The Essential Diabetic Cookbook

The Essential Diabetic Cookbook

A comprehensive guide to diet and diabetes with a selection of high-fibre, low-fat and low-sugar recipes

Azmina Govindji and Jill Myers

Thorsons
An Imprint of HarperCollins*Publishers*

Thorsons
An Imprint of HarperCollins*Publishers*
77–85 Fulham Palace Road,
Hammersmith, London W6 8JB

Published by Thorsons 1992
1   3   5   7   9   10   8   6   4   2

A catalogue record for this book
is available from the British Library

ISBN 0 7225 2505 2

Typeset by Harper Phototypesetters Limited,
Northampton, England
Printed in Great Britain by
The Bath Press, Bath, Avon

Contents

Acknowledgements

The authors would like to thank the following people for their patience and invaluable help: Georgina West for typing the recipes; Sue Brenchley, Stella Bowling, Jane Bebell, Sue Bosanko and Judith North for their valuable comments; and Anise Kanji and Hanif Ladha for typing the text.

And thanks to our husbands for being so tolerant!

Foreword

Food is one of life's great pleasures. Having diabetes does not and need not change that. People with diabetes should know that they can enjoy any food they want. They must bear in mind just two constraints — quantity and timing.

Diabetes is having too little insulin action and, therefore, too much sugar. Food and insulin are closely linked. When the person without diabetes eats a meal, the pancreas gland automatically delivers into the bloodstream just enough insulin to process the foodstuffs for the body. People with diabetes can no longer do this. They need an 'insulin assist'. Some may be able to boost their own diminished insulin supply with a tablet, while others produce so little that they have to inject it from a syringe.

For people injecting insulin, the dose and meal need to be in balance to control and prevent wide swings — upwards or downwards — of the amount of glucose in the blood. Often, the insulin is injected just before the meal so that the two meet together. With tablets the link is not quite so close, but meal timing is important to prevent the blood glucose falling to very low levels (hypoglycaemia). For overweight people, the dietitian will advise a reducing diet — all the foods but less of them.

All this must sound complicated, even menacing to the newly diagnosed diabetic — not exactly a prescription for carefree mealtime enjoyment. However, once the initial shock has passed, a few simple facts absorbed and confidence restored, normal food and interesting meals are emphatically back on the agenda. That's when *The Essential Diabetic Cookbook* comes into play. It is full of delicious dishes, aromatic advice, mouthwatering morsels. At the same time, it is a painless guide to healthy and hearty eating for the whole family.

The two authors of the book, Azmina Govindji and Jill Myers, are both very experienced in their fields. Azmina Govindji, Chief Dietitian of the British Diabetic Association, has been actively involved in the development of guidelines for diet in diabetes since 1987. As Head of the Diet Information Service, she maintains close links with government bodies, academic institutions, health professionals, food manufacturers and the media. Azmina offers advice on all matters relating to food and diabetes.

Jill Myers, formerly Home Economist to the British Diabetic Association, has considerable experience in recipe development and cookery demonstrations. While at the Association she was responsible for the production of a range of tried and tested recipes for people with diabetes and for catering establishments. She was the primary source of advice on recipe modification. Jill Myers is now working for a major food retailer as a home economist developing quality own label ambient ready meals.

Whether you cook it or just eat it, with the help of this book you can look forward to pleasurable culinary ventures and enjoyable mealtimes. So, read on and *bon appetit!*

Professor Harry Keen, MD, FRCP
Chairman, Executive Council,
British Diabetic Association,
Professor Emeritus, United Medical
and Dental School, Guy's Hospital Campus

What's so special about this book?

You may never need another cookbook. Why not? Because this book tells you all you need to know about food now that you have diabetes. It is not just another cookery publication. This book

- is the most up-to-date cookery book for people with diabetes, incorporating all the latest dietary policies from the British Diabetic Association
- contains a wide variety of high-fibre, low-fat, low-sugar recipes that are in line with the general principles of healthy eating. This means it provides attractive recipes and essential information not only for people with diabetes, but also for anyone wishing to lose weight or to eat more healthily
- has something for everyone — the elderly who need to prepare quick, easy, and possibly cheap meals; students living on limited budgets; parents who want to provide nutritious food for the family; the keen cook who invites guests with diabetes to dinner; vegetarians and vegans; the weight watcher; and, of course, the person with diabetes
- is a comprehensive guide to diabetes and its dietary treatment.

Sections include information on choosing the right mix of foods, healthy eating for the whole family, watching your weight, eating out, what to do in an emergency and lots more. Then there are over 200 recipes to help you put it all into practice. From soups and starters to tasty meat, fish and vegetarian dishes, this book is a must for anyone who wants to cook everyday food in an appetizing way. And who said people with diabetes shouldn't eat puddings? The mouth-watering pudding and dessert recipes will certainly prove that you need not compromise on taste just because you have diabetes!

Introducing diabetes

What is diabetes?

Diabetes mellitus (commonly known as diabetes) affects about two per cent of the UK population, and over 30 million people worldwide. In people with diabetes, the glucose (sugar) level in the blood is too high because the mechanism that converts sugar to energy no longer works properly. Glucose is normally carried by the blood to the body's cells (a cell is the basic structural unit of the body). With the help of a hormone called insulin, the glucose enters the cells and is used to provide the body's energy. If there is not enough insulin in the body, or if the body cannot make effective use of what insulin there is, then the glucose cannot enter the cells. As a result sugar builds up in the bloodstream, causing diabetes. Symptoms of diabetes include needing to pass water (urinate) very frequently, increased thirst, hunger, weight loss, tiredness, itching of the genital organs and blurring of vision.

There are two main types of diabetes: insulin dependent diabetes (IDDM) and non-insulin dependent diabetes (NIDDM). IDDM affects approximately one quarter of the people who have diabetes. It generally occurs in young people, and treatment consists of insulin injections with an appropriate food plan. NIDDM usually occurs in middle-aged and older people and often in those who are overweight. It is treated by a modified diet, and drugs may also be used. The two main aims of treatment are to eliminate the symptoms and to prevent long-term complications, such as eye, nerve, kidney and foot problems.

Diet is the foundation for the management of diabetes and the control of symptoms, and following a sensible food plan will help to keep your blood sugar close to the normal range. The diet for diabetes is not a special one in any way: it is a healthy eating pattern which is recommended for everyone, with or without diabetes, and one that the whole family can enjoy. The information in this book covers the basic aspects of the dietary recommendations for diabetes. Further help with your diabetes is available from your local Diabetic Association (see Useful addresses, on page 197).

Don't worry if all you've heard about eating well is that carrots help you see better in the dark and spinach gives you iron — just read on.

If you have diabetes, remember to:

- continue with your treatment even if symptoms have disappeared
- attend the clinic for regular check-ups.

Your feelings

Being told that you have a condition which will last for the rest of your life is bound to have an effect on how you organize the practical aspects of daily living and also on your feelings. It is natural for you, your family and your friends to feel sad about the loss of spontaneity that diabetes can sometimes cause. Perhaps you feel angry, asking yourself, 'Why me?' and maybe you are worried about the future.

At times like this, talking to other people who also live with diabetes can be a great help. They can share their experiences with you and give you support. The team at your diabetes clinic may be able to put you in contact with other people with diabetes. Also, your local Diabetic Association will know people who you can contact and may also arrange local support groups.

Diabetes isn't all bad. There are people with diabetes in all walks of life — from professional sports people to politicians. Some of them will work in occupations or follow interests *you* want to pursue. Although you will have to think ahead a little more than you did before, don't feel that having diabetes prevents you from having a full life.

Healthy eating

Why is is to important to eat healthily? Research studies worldwide suggest that watching what you eat is not only essential to the management of diabetes, but that it can also help prevent heart disease, constipation, bowel problems, obesity and tooth decay. Following a good diet also makes you feel good!

There is no such thing as a bad food; there is only a bad diet. All foods can have some nutritional benefit, but it is the mix of foods and the amounts you eat that make what you eat healthy or unhealthy.

In diabetes, the nutrient value of a food is not the only consideration. The way a particular food is digested and its effect on blood sugar can influence the general control of diabetes. For example, mashed potatoes can make blood sugar rise quicker than the same amount of boiled potatoes, simply because vegetables that are left whole take longer to digest. Other factors can also make a difference to blood sugar levels. Because of this, it is difficult to arrange foods into 'goods, bads, and mediums'. However, Tables 1 and 2 will give you some idea about which foods to choose or avoid.

Table 1 *Foods that can be eaten freely*

Vegetables

Cauliflower	Salad vegetables	Tomatoes
Runner beans	Marrow	Peppers
Carrots	Mushrooms	Swede
All green leafy vegetables	Celery	Turnip
Frozen and fresh peas	Onions	

Fruit

Cranberries	Lemons	Redcurrants
Gooseberries	Loganberries	
Grapefruit	Rhubarb	

Beverages

Tea	Soda water	
Coffee	Lemon juice	
Sugar-free squashes and	Tomato juice	
mixers	Clear soups	

Seasonings

Pepper	Pickles	Spices
Mustard	Herbs	Stock cubes
Vinegar	Essences	Food colourings

Table 2 *Foods to restrict your consumption of*

Marmalade*, jam*, honey*, lemon curd
Mincemeat
Syrup, treacle
Sugar
Glucose
Glucose tablets
Fizzy and mixer drinks*, cordial*, squashes*
Sweet pastries and cakes
Fruit tinned in syrup*

* Low-sugar or sugar-free alternatives to these items are available.

The foods in table 2 are high in sugar and have virtually no nutritional value.

The following general guidelines on healthy eating will also help you to choose the right types of food. You don't need to do everything at once; start by choosing those ideas you find the easiest and gradually try to bring in the others.

- Cut down on fat and fatty foods.
- Eat more fibre-rich foods.
- Eat less sugar.
- Cut down on salt.
- Go easy on alcohol.

Introducing diabetes

The following suggestions will help you to implement these guidelines, while the recipes in this book will enable you to prepare your favourite foods in a healthier way. Eating a variety of healthy foods can give you a sense of well-being and vitality.

Fat

A high fat intake has been shown to increase your chances of becoming obese (very overweight) or of developing heart disease. It therefore makes sense to cut down on the amount of fatty foods you eat regardless of whether or not you have diabetes. There are three main types of fat:

- saturated fats, such as dairy products, animal fats
- polyunsaturated fats, such as corn oil, sunflower oil, fish oil
- monounsaturated fats, such as olive oil, rapeseed oil, peanut oil.

Cholesterol

Cholesterol is a fatty substance that forms an essential part of the body's cells, but, equally, too much cholesterol in the body can cause problems. If the level of cholesterol in your blood is too high, you increase your chances of developing heart disease. Cholesterol can build up in the arteries (the large blood vessels) in the heart. This accumulation of cholesterol can eventually cause the arteries to become completely blocked, leading to a heart attack.

Some foods are high in cholesterol, but cutting down on these alone does not make a significant difference to blood cholesterol levels. It is more important that you cut down on the amount of *saturated* fat that you eat, as eating too much saturated fat increases your blood cholesterol level. This is particularly important for people with diabetes, as they are more prone to heart problems.

The unsaturated fats do not raise blood cholesterol in the same way that saturated fats do. Evidence now suggests that monounsaturated fats can also help keep blood cholesterol levels low. A lot of monounsaturated fat in the form of olive oil is eaten in the traditional diets of most Mediterranean countries and the rate of heart disease in these countries is low, so it would seem that the diet may be one of the factors responsible for this. Studies in other countries have also shown that healthy diets low in saturated fat and high in monounsaturated fat may reduce the risk of developing heart disease. There seems, therefore, to be an advantage in substituting foods that are high in saturated fat with polyunsaturated and monounsaturated alternatives, as well as reducing your total fat intake.

> Remember that *all* fats and oils are high in calories, so use only small quantities and choose monounsaturated or poly-unsaturated types whenever possible.

Fish oils

Rates of heart disease are also low in countries where fish are eaten in large quantities. It is thought that this is because of a particular type of fat contained in fish oils. It has not yet been absolutely proved, but you certainly have nothing to lose by eating more fish. Oily fish such as mackerel, herring, salmon and trout are an excellent source of protein and of vitamins A, D and E. Try to replace some of your meat intake with fish (especially oily fish) to improve the overall quality of your diet while helping you to cut down on your total fat intake. How about making Mackerel in Cider Sauce (see page 84) or Smoked Mackerel Pâté (see page 46).

Fats and figures

Remember that fat is a very concentrated source of calories, so eating less fat can help you lose weight. (Calories are units used to measure the energy values of foods — see Counting Calories on page 29 for more information). One boiled egg is approximately 70 kcalories. Have it fried and the calories almost double. A tablespoon of oil is approximately 100 kcalories — this is about the same number of calories as half a pint of beer. Think about this when you see an oily dressing on a salad!

Low-fat foods can play an important role in reducing the total amount of fat in your diet. Whether you are watching your weight, need to eat less for a specific medical condition or are simply trying to avoid a heart attack, low-fat foods can make life much easier. However, be careful not to rely too heavily on some of them (such as low-fat sausages, low-fat cream cheese, low-fat crisps) because they still provide a lot of calories. Furthermore, low-fat spreads are not fat-free, so don't use twice as much!

How to eat less fat

- Avoid frying foods — grill, bake, boil, poach or steam instead.
- Butter and all margarines contain about the same amount of fat. Choose a polyunsaturated margarine and spread thinly or try a reduced or low-fat polyunsaturated or monounsaturated spread. Ordinary low-fat spreads are also a good substitute for butter.
- Use lower fat versions of dairy products, for example, semi-skimmed or skimmed milk, half-fat cheddar, cottage cheese, low-fat yogurt.
- Cut down on fat-containing snack foods such as crisps, cakes, chocolates and biscuits.
- Buy lean meat or trim the fat off fatty meat. Poultry can be low in fat if the skin is removed. Eat fish more often. Oily fish is high in polyunsaturated fat, but, remember, do not fry it!
- Watch out for processed foods that are high in fat, such as pies and other meat products — read the label.
- If you do use oil in cooking, use as little as possible. Choose one that is high in polyunsaturated fat (such as corn oil, sunflower oil, safflower oil, soya oil) or monounsaturated fat (such as olive oil, rapeseed oil, peanut oil). Experiment with using olive oil by trying the Courgette and Sweetcorn Gratin (see page 109) or Red Lentil Lasagne (see page 98) recipes.

Introducing diabetes

All the recipes in this book encourage low-fat cooking methods.

Fibre

Fibre-rich foods are important to the prevention and treatment of constipation. Also, being filling and generally low in calories, they are useful if you are trying to lose weight as you feel full after eating less.

In diabetes, foods high in a particular type of fibre — soluble fibre — can improve blood glucose (sugar) control. Research has shown that the soluble fibre found in oats, beans and lentils can slow down the rise in blood glucose levels after a meal, so it makes sense for people with diabetes to eat these foods frequently. Soluble fibre can also reduce abnormally high blood cholesterol. Some of the recipes that follow, such as the Chick Pea Moussaka (see page 000), demonstrate how you can use such foods to cook a substantial and appetizing meal.

> Current nutritional thinking recommends that everyone include more fibre in their diet.

When you increase your intake of fibre, do so gradually: a new style of eating should never be adopted in haste. Drink more fluids, too, in the form of water or low-calorie drinks because your body needs plenty of fluid to digest fibrous foods.

Ways of eating more fibre

- Choose wholemeal, wholegrain or granary bread, vegetables with a skin (such as jacket potatoes, sweetcorn, peas), beans, lentils, brown rice and high-fibre breakfast cereals (such as porridge, muesli, bran-based cereals) in preference to more refined low-fibre foods.
- Substitute fruit juice with fresh fruit (a glass of apple juice has around 100 kcalories and no fibre whereas an apple provides only about 40 kcalories and has 2 grams of fibre).
- Choose foods as close to their natural state as possible. A food that is refined or processed generally contains less fibre. For example, white flour is lower in fibre than wholemeal flour, which has been made from the whole of the wheat grain.
- Keep high-fibre foods as whole as possible, having boiled or baked potatoes rather than mashed, and make a whole bean casserole (such as the Mixed Bean Hot Pot on page 105) instead of a puréed lentil soup. Such foods are digested more slowly and this helps to keep blood sugar levels steady.
- Try to use more beans, peas and lentils. They are cheaper than meat and are a good source of protein and fibre. Tinned baked beans are a quick way of

getting more fibre and you don't even need to buy the sugar-free variety — the ordinary ones contain an insignificant amount of sugar.

Sugar

It is often thought that sugar is needed for energy. However, energy is also derived from starch, protein and fat — in fact, every type of food we eat provides us with energy. All we get from sugar is calories. Sugar contains no useful nutrients nor has it any special energy-giving properties over other foods. In people with diabetes, sugary foods can cause blood glucose to rise rapidly, which is undesirable. Sugary foods can also lead to tooth decay, particularly if they are eaten between meals. Also, as sugar-containing foods are often high in fat and low in fibre, eating too many chocolates, desserts and cakes can make you put on weight.

Much of the sugar we eat is added by food manufacturers. Some packaged foods may be high in sugar even when they appear to be healthy, such as cakes and biscuits bought from health food shops. The ingredients list may not even specify sugar — but watch out for words like maltose, dextrose, honey, treacle, golden syrup, fructose, and corn syrup on the label. All of these are types of sugar and are not significantly better for you than sugar. Remember, too, that sucrose is simply the chemical term for ordinary, white table sugar.

Get into the habit of reading labels and choosing foods that are low in *all* forms of sugar. If an item is low down on the ingredients list, there is less of that ingredient in the food than the ingredients given before it.

Sugar can cause tooth decay and eating too many sugary foods can make you put on weight, so eat less sugar.

Sugar and diabetes — putting it into context

People with diabetes are advised to avoid drinks containing sugar. Because the sugar in these drinks is in liquid form, it can enter the blood quite quickly. This causes blood sugar to rise rapidly. With diabetes, you want to avoid this.

However, if sugar is taken mixed in with food (such as an ice-cream after a meal), then blood sugar rises more slowly. So, if you wish to eat a small amount of sweet food, such as a piece of cake or a dessert, then try to have it after a meal.

Cutting down on sugar

- Try not to add sugar to drinks or cereals. There is a range of artificial sweeteners that make excellent substitutes (see Artificial Sweeteners, page 22).
- Choose unsweetened fruit juice, and diet or low-calorie drinks rather than sweetened soft drinks. One 330ml can of a sweetened fizzy drink can contain 7 teaspoons of sugar!
- Buy reduced-sugar jams, pure fruit spreads and fruit tinned in natural juice instead of their sweetened alternatives.

Introducing diabetes

- Save cakes, sweets and chocolates for special occasions only.
- Look at labels and try to avoid manufactured foods that contain a lot of sugar.

What about fructose?

Recipes for people with diabetes have traditionally used fructose (fruit sugar). However, after an extensive review of the studies conducted on sucrose (ordinary sugar), the British Diabetic Association now recommends that a small amount of sucrose is perfectly acceptable in home baking, provided that it is mixed with high-fibre ingredients and eaten as part of a healthy diet. The Nutrition Study Group of the European Association for the Study of Diabetes and the Australian Diabetes Association have similar recommendations on sucrose. The American Diabetes Association states that small amounts of sucrose may be acceptable for people who are not overweight, provided that the diabetes is well controlled.

The recipes in this book also follow these recommendations, containing ordinary sugar together with high-fibre ingredients. This not only makes them more appealing to the whole family, but also makes them more affordable, as ordinary sugar costs less than fructose. Of course, sugar has only been used in recipes where an artificial sweetener cannot be used instead.

Salt

Most experts on nutrition advise you to eat less salt. Why?

In some people, eating salt may be linked with high blood pressure. Although a small amount of salt is needed by the body, it is possible for the average person to eat up to ten times more salt than the body requires. A lot of the salt we eat is added by the manufacturers during food processing. Cutting down on processed food can therefore help you to eat less salt.

Cutting down on salt

- Use less salt in cooking (experiment with other seasonings, such as herbs and spices).
- Avoid adding salt at the table.
- Eat fewer salty manufactured foods, such as smoked and preserved meat and fish, sausages and salted snack foods.

Alcohol

Weight for weight, alcohol contains more calories than sugar, so even moderate drinking can make you gain weight. For example, one pint of beer has about the same number of calories as three chocolate biscuits. Also, as alcohol contains negligible nutrients, it is of little dietary benefit. Replacing meals with alcoholic drinks can make you lose out on important vitamins and minerals. If you have diabetes, you don't need to give up drinking alcohol altogether, but you do need to think more carefully about what you drink and when.

Alcohol in large quantities can damage your liver. The recommended maximum intake

These drinks all contain roughly the same amount of alcohol.

½ pint ordinary beer	=	*single measure of spirits	=	small glass of sherry	=	glass of wine	=	1 unit

*In Northern Ireland a single measure of spirits = 1½ units.

for anyone, with or without diabetes, is 3 units of alcohol for men and 2 units for women. Try to have two or three drink-free days each week. Pregnant and breastfeeding women should ideally avoid alcoholic drinks altogether.

The above all contain one unit of alcohol.

Use the guidelines below to help you keep your social drinking to safe limits.

- Do not exceed the recommended maximum intakes.
- Try low-sugar, low-alcohol drinks — they are better for your blood glucose (important if you have diabetes) and for your waistline.
- Never drink on an empty stomach; eat before you drink.

- Alternate your alcoholic drinks with alcohol-free drinks. If drinking spirits, use sugar-free mixers or soda water.
- Remember not to drink and drive.
- If you have diabetes, you should also note the following:
  - you may drink up to three units of sweet wine or sherry as part of your weekly allowance, but try not to drink them all on the same occasion
  - you should avoid the special low-carbohydrate beers and lagers that were originally brewed for people with diabetes — they are higher in alcohol and calories than ordinary beers
  - it is important to wear some form of diabetic identification — you and others may confuse low blood sugar

Introducing diabetes

(hypoglycaemia) with drunkenness
- alcohol lowers blood sugar, so remember this, particularly if you are on insulin. This (hypoglycaemic) effect can last several hours.
- if you count how much carbohydrate (CHO) you eat, don't include the CHO from alcoholic drinks.

Artificial sweeteners — not sugar, but sweet

Artificial sweeteners have made an enormous range of foods readily available for all those who want to avoid large quantities of sugar — slimmers, the health conscious and people with diabetes. They impart an intense level of sweetness and are virtually calorie-free. Available as tablets, liquids or in granulated form, they can be used to replace sugar in drinks, cereals and puddings. They are also found in many reduced-calorie foods such as diet yogurts, low-calorie squash and diet soft drinks.

All these artificial substitutes for sugar are food additives and so are required by law to undergo rigorous tests for safety before being approved for use. Examples of those commonly used are aspartame, saccharin, and acesulfame potassium (acesulfame K). All of these are widely available under various brand names. Neohesperidine (NHDC) is the newest permitted sweetener in this country. Cyclamate is widely sold in Europe and may receive approval for sale in the UK.

Personal preferences vary, so it is a good idea to shop around until you find one that suits your palate and your pocket best — the prices also vary! If you tend to use a lot of sweeteners in drinks, cereals, puddings and processed foods, make sure you vary the type of sweetener you choose so as to reduce any chance of over-consumption of one food additive.

Unlike sugar, artificial sweeteners do not cause tooth decay and are virtually calorie-free.

Diabetic products

These specialist products have been on the market since the 1960s. At that time, the diabetic diet strictly prohibited the consumption of sugar and a low carbohydrate intake was encouraged. Because of this, special diabetic foods that were sugar-free and low in carbohydrate were considered to be a good idea.

Times change, however, and, as we learn more about nutrition, so do recommended diets. Today a high-carbohydrate, high-fibre diet is recommended and a small amount of sugar is acceptable, provided that it forms part of this diet. So treats can now include ordinary chocolates, cakes or biscuits, so long as they are eaten in small amounts within the context of a healthy diet, preferably at the end of a meal. Useful proprietary products that are not marketed especially for people with diabetes are sugar-free drinks, diet yogurts and artificial sweeteners.

So, you don't *need* to buy or eat special diabetic products. Because they are also expensive and are often no lower in fat or calories than their non-diabetic equivalents, consuming them is now discouraged in many countries.

Making meals

You now know which foods are the better ones to choose and which foods to cut down on; you will shortly learn which cooking methods to adopt and have a selection of tasty recipes, but how do you transform all this knowledge and information into practical food terms? How do you 'make meals'?

Here is an example of a day's food intake. Have a go at changing the foods chosen and the cooking methods so that the meals are healthier and more appropriate for people with diabetes. Then turn the page to find a possible solution — see how your suggestions compare.

A day's food	Healthier choices
Breakfast	
Cornflakes with whole milk and sugar	
White toast with butter and jam	
Coffee with milk and sugar	
Lunch	
2 slices white bread with Cheddar cheese, tomato and mayonnaise	
Banana	
Sugary fizzy drink, such as Coke	
Mid-afternoon snack	
2 chocolate biscuits	
Tea with milk and sugar	
Supper	
Shepherd's pie	
Cabbage	
Fruit crumble	
Custard	
Bedtime	
Tea with milk and sugar	

Introducing diabetes

Healthier choices	Comments
Breakfast	
Breakfast cereal containing bran or porridge or muesli	• more fibre • oats contain soluble fibre
Semi-skimmed or skimmed milk	• less fat
Granulated artificial sweetener	• sugar free
Wholemeal or granary toast	• whole grains may help keep blood sugar at a safe level
Polyunsaturated or monounsaturated margarine or low-fat spread	• less saturated fat • less total fat and fewer calories
Reduced-sugar jam or	• less sugar
pure fruit spread	• fewer calories
Coffee with semi-skimmed or skimmed milk	• less fat
Artificial sweetener	• sugar free
Lunch	
2 slices wholemeal or granary bread	• more fibre
Low-fat or half-fat cheddar or cottage cheese or Edam cheese	• less fat
Tomato	
Reduced-calorie mayonnaise	• less fat and fewer calories
Banana	
Diet fizzy drink (such as diet Coke or equivalent)	• sugar free and fewer calories
Mid-afternoon snack	
2 plain biscuits	• less sugar, less fat and fewer calories
Tea with semi-skimmed or skimmed milk	• less fat and fewer calories
Artificial sweetener	• sugar free

Healthier choices	Comments
Supper	
Lean savoury mince	• less fat
Boiled or baked potatoes in	• more fibre
their jackets	• vegetables kept whole
Sweetcorn	• more soluble fibre
Fruit crumble, sweetened with	
artificial sweetener and	• sugar free
crumble topping made from	
wholemeal flour, muesli, poly- or	• more fibre (muesli has soluble fibre)
monounsaturated margarine or	• less saturated fat or less total fat
low-fat spread	
Bedtime	
Tea with semi-skimmed or skimmed milk	• less fat
Artificial sweetener	• sugar free

As you can see, only small changes have been made, but by choosing low-fat, high-fibre, low-sugar foods and by adopting sensible cooking methods, the health giving quality of the meals has been greatly improved. Use this guide and the practical cooking tips on page 37 to help you make all your meals more healthy.

Eating away from home

If you have diabetes, there is no reason why you can't visit the local fast food joint, the posh restaurant in town, go to your friend's house for dinner or a holiday resort abroad.

A quick take-away

As with any food or drink, it makes sense to limit the amount of 'fast food' you eat. It does have the benefit of being quick and convenient, so avoiding it altogether can be a nuisance. Simply try not to rely on such foods too often and, when you do, make the most healthy choice possible. For example, choose a smaller hamburger in a wholemeal bun, if available, and unsweetened orange juice or a diet drink. Try to resist that sugary, processed apple pie. They are often more like apple fritters than pies and can be incredibly high in fat. Remember, too, that one milkshake can have more calories than seven wine glasses of fresh orange juice!

The Chinese stir-fry is becoming an increasingly popular fast-food choice. These foods are generally healthy, particularly since a wide variety of vegetables make up an important part of the meal. Obviously the oily dishes such as deep fried seaweed, spring rolls, fried prawn balls, crispy Peking duck and fried noodles can be very high in fat, and steamed alternatives are preferable. The main meals generally contain very little carbohydrate and only the rice and noodle dishes need to be counted if you are on a daily carbohydrate allowance. Sweet and sour dishes are best kept for special occasions. They tend to be high in fat, sugar and calories.

The Greek doner kebab may look lean, but have you noticed the oil that trickles down the outside? Don't believe you have lost all of the fat in this way, there is still 'hidden' fat in the meat. Lower fat choices are grilled kebabs, especially chicken. Fill some hot pitta bread (preferably wholemeal) with kebabs and a colourful salad for a filling, nutritious and convenient meal.

The local 'chippy' unfortunately does not have many healthy foods on offer since most items are deep fried or contain pastry. Ordering a couple of rolls and less of the fatty food can be helpful.

The tempting aroma emanating from an Indian restaurant can act like a magnet when you are hungry! Choose lentil (or dahl) based dishes, tandooris and grills, naan or chapati (unbuttered) and boiled rice. Save high fat dishes like fried poppadums, butter chicken, paratha (deep fried Indian bread) and biryani or pilau rice for special occasions. Did you know that an average portion of pilau rice has more than double the calories of a portion of plain boiled rice?

Dining in style

What about a night out at an exclusive restaurant? On a special occasion, why not enjoy yourself and eat what you like? If it is your birthday, anniversary, Christmas, whatever, do you think it will do you much harm to forget the fat and fibre for just one evening? If you want a small serving of dessert, remember that sugar has a less drastic effect on your blood sugar level when it mixed in with lots of other ingredients and eaten at the end of a meal. (Remember if you take insulin, though, that you may need to make some adjustments — see page 27).

If you eat out frequently, however, perhaps attending business lunches or spending three nights a week wining and dining, then you need to think more carefully about the foods you choose. Try to avoid rich, creamy sauces, fried foods and sweet, fattening desserts. Watch the amount of alcohol you have, too.

Guess who's coming to dinner?

When a friend invites you to dinner, don't forget that other people's knowledge of diabetes and food may be limited. If you feel that you would like to plan ahead, it may be worth letting your host or hostess know which foods you would prefer to be served — perhaps some of the mouthwatering dishes from this book! Otherwise, simply select whatever you think best from the dining table and, remember, an occasional lapse from your diet is not detrimental.

Sun, sand, sea — and food

A little thoughtful planning before setting off for a week in the sun can make an important difference to your trip. Many people nowadays prefer self-catering accommodation, which will obviously mean that you have maximum control over what you eat. However, hotels often have a reasonable choice on the menu. If you are confronted with a range of unusual foods you are not sure about, you can almost always ask for bread, pasta or rice with a simple accompaniment like an omelette or cheese until you have discovered exactly what is on offer.

Remember to take extra carbohydrate supplies with you on the journey to your holiday destination. Suitable convenience snacks include sandwiches, fruit, biscuits and crisps. Take emergency supplies of glucose tablets or sweets along as well.

Insulin and carbohydrate when eating out

If you take insulin, adjustments may need to be made to:

- your preceding snack or meal
- your insulin dose
- the timing of your injection.

You will probably work out what sort of changes are required by trial and error, but the following tips may be useful:

- plan ahead whenever possible
- extra carbohydrate (CHO) does need extra insulin (the dose depends on how much CHO is in the food)
- extra insulin is usually taken in the form of a quick-acting insulin shortly before a meal — this is particularly helpful if the meal is served later than you had anticipated
- you could delay the timing of your insulin injection if your meal is due to be taken later than usual
- if you are eating late, you could try having a snack at your usual mealtime to prevent your blood sugar from falling too low before your main meal
- if you use a pen injector, you will have a greater degree of flexibility — you can assess the CHO value of your meal and inject accordingly
- if you are dining and dancing, remember that the energy you use up while dancing will lower your blood sugar and, consequently, you may need to inject less insulin or eat more carbohydrate
- alcohol lowers blood sugar. Normally this is not a problem, but if you take insulin, it is important to have some food before or with an alcoholic drink and, most importantly, afterwards (such as a bedtime snack). This will prevent your blood sugar level falling too low, as the effect of alcohol can last for several hours.

Emergency measures for low blood sugar

The medical term for a low blood sugar level is hypoglycaemia or a hypo. Hypos are most likely to occur in people who inject insulin, but some people on certain tablets may also experience a hypo. It can be caused by:

- missing a meal or snack
- eating less carbohydrate than usual
- engaging in strenuous activity that you have not compensated for by, for example, eating some carbohydrate
- injecting more insulin than you need
- drinking alcohol on an empty stomach.

Please don't feel that you have to look for a cause, however, as there may be no obvious reason.

Signs and symptoms of hypoglycaemia vary from one person to the next, but common ones include light-headedness, a faint feeling, sweating, shaking, hunger and confusion. You will soon learn the warning signs of a hypo and it is a good idea to let a friend or relative know what these are, too, so that they can recognize one.

What to do if you have a hypo

The main aim is to raise your blood sugar level quickly. The fastest way to do this is to have some form of concentrated sugar (see the list below for examples) immediately, followed by a snack, such as a slice of bread, biscuits or milk.

Carry something from the list below with you at all times. Wearing some sort of diabetic identification is an effective way of telling people you don't know around you that you have diabetes, should you need further help in such instances. If you cannot swallow, a doctor or ambulance should be called immediately. If you know why the hypo occurred, try to make adjustments to prevent it happening again. Seek the advice of your doctor, diabetes specialist nurse or dietitian if necessary.

Illness

When you are ill, you may not feel like eating. However, even if you do not eat any food, you will find that your blood sugar level tends to go up when you are ill. Your body naturally responds to illness by making more sugar. It is obviously very important, therefore, to *continue with your diabetic treatment*. The following suggestions may also be useful:

- consult your doctor, particularly if you are vomiting
- if you are not eating, take fluids such as fruit juice, soup or a glucose drink (such as Lucozade), with 'a little and often', being a good motto — for example, half a glass every hour

Suggested emergency items	Amount to take
Glucose tablets	3 tablets
Sugar or glucose powder	2 teaspoons
Sugar cubes	2 cubes
Sweets and candies	3 sweets
Honey, jam or syrup	2 teaspoons
Lucozade or similar glucose drink	50ml (2 fl oz)
Sugared fizzy drink, such as ordinary coca-cola	½ glass
Orange juice	½ glass

- if you are eating, have small, frequent meals
- if possible, test your blood sugar or urine at least four times a day and keep a record of the results
- if you take insulin, the dose may need adjusting — for example, if your blood sugar is very high, you will need more insulin (call your doctor if you need help with this)
- if you have a temperature, take two paracetamol tablets four times a day — do not take aspirin without your doctor's permission as it can have an effect on your diabetes medication.

Counting calories

What are calories?

The term 'calories' or 'kcalories' (kilocalories) is used to describe the amount of energy provided by the food you eat. All food provides calories but some foods are more concentrated in calories than others. For example, a 100 g (4 oz) apple will provide you with around 50 kcalories, whereas a 100 g (4 oz) piece of Cheddar cheese would provide 400 kcalories. This is because every food contains a different proportion of fat, carbohydrate and protein. Weight for weight, fat contains twice as many calories as either carbohydrate or protein. Therefore, those foods that have a higher percentage of fat are likely to be highest in calories.

On food labels, the calorific value of a food is usually written as kcal/100g. For example, if a label states 350 kcals/100g then this means that a 100 g (4 oz) portion of the food would provide 350 kcalories. You may also see the term kilojoule (kj) used on labels. One kcalorie is equal to 4.2kj.

If the number of calories you take in from the food you eat is the *same* as the number you use up in your daily activities, your weight should be more less stable. However, if you take in *more* calories from food than you use up, you are likely to gain weight. On the other hand, if you eat *less* than normal but maintain your usual level of activity, you may lose weight.

Why count calories?

Being overweight can increase your chances of developing diabetes, heart disease and high blood pressure. If you have diabetes and are overweight, weight reduction can improve the control of your diabetes and may even mean that you can reduce the dosage of your medication.

Motivation

Why is it that at some time in their lives most people have tried some sort of slimming diet, that the bookshops are oozing with novel ideas on how to shed those extra pounds and yet obesity is *still* a major problem in most Western countries?

From the restricted grapefruit diet (very silly and not to be encouraged) to the more sensible high-fibre, low-fat type of diet, you are presented with hundreds of ways to cut down on calories. Often one of these will help you lose weight but, more often than not, the weight starts to creep back on again. There are, no doubt, many reasons for this, but one of the most important is motivation — or lack of it. If you can maintain

Introducing diabetes

your motivation, then you are more likely to make a concerted effort to persevere. How, though, can you keep yourself motivated? It is unlikely that you will keep to a diet if it makes unreasonable demands on your normal lifestyle. Only if your new way of eating fits in with your social habits, your time constraints, your budget and your food preferences will you have a strong chance of keeping your weight down for a significant length of time.

Support

Reputable commercial slimming clubs can provide invaluable personal support as you try to lose weight. Most people who are trying to lose weight need guidance on more than just what to put on their plates at mealtimes. Psychological and emotional support can make changing your eating behaviour much easier and often these clubs can provide a degree of one-to-one counselling.

In some cases, your doctor may refer you to the dietitian at the local hospital or clinic. A qualified dietitian will take your medical history, age, sex and lifestyle into account and will then be able to help you with a personal food plan. Men often lose weight on 1200-1500 kcalories per day, while women are usually advised to keep to 1000-1200 kcalories per day. However, this can vary from person to person. The dietitian can, in addition, offer guidance and support as necessary.

If you follow the general guidelines on Healthy eating given on pages 14-16 you will be able to adopt a style of eating that will help you lose weight while still providing you with all the nutrients you need. If you choose the foods you eat sensibly and cook them in the ways suggested in this book, you will be able to reduce your calorie intake and still enjoy tasty, filling meals.

Sensible slimming suggestions

- Be realistic when deciding how much weight you want to lose — setting a goal that seems unattainable could make you feel frustrated and give up.
- Set short-term targets and reward yourself once you've reached them. For example, treat yourself to a record or a book after you've lost 7lb (about 3kg). Don't use food as a reward, though, or you'll undo all your good work!
- Try recording *exactly* what you eat — you may be surprised to see how the nibbles and snacks mount up.
- Make changes slowly. For example, try to avoid fried foods one week and, then, in the following week, to eat high-fibre breakfast cereals as well.
- Write down your successes — this can help keep you motivated.
- Try to encourage your family to eat healthily. This way you won't need to prepare foods specifically for yourself, you will simply need to have smaller portions.
- Think of ways to help your meals appear larger. Use a smaller plate, or have a selection of vegetables.

- Try to avoid TV dinners as concentrating on TV can make you less aware of how much you're eating. Try to sit down when you are eating — it's amazing how much you can munch your way through on the move!
- Don't shop when you're hungry — you may be tempted into buying more than you need (using a shopping list is a good idea) and avoid the aisles full of sweets and biscuits and the cakes at the in-store bakery!

As time goes on your body adapts to your new calorie intake by needing fewer calories for normal functions such as breathing. Don't be discouraged, keep at it. Keep up the motivation, maintain variety, experiment with new recipes, reward yourself (but not with food) when you have done well, exercise, eat out (sensibly) on occasions, take up a new hobby, diet with a friend or whatever else helps. Do everything within your power to get down to that target weight — it will be worth it.

Are you overweight?

It's obviously worth finding out if you *need* to lose weight before you start slimming. Use the chart overleaf to estimate how much (if any) weight you need to lose. Remember not to make unreasonable demands on yourself. Aim to get down to a weight that is practical and possible. Don't bother to weigh yourself every day as you may find you lose one day and gain the next. This is normal, but can be disheartening. Try to weigh yourself only once a week and at around the same time of day.

Diets that offer a weight loss of 7lb (3kg) in a week may sound like a miracle cure, but will not help you in the long term. So be patient — it took time to gain the excess weight, so losing it effectively is going to take time, too. The ideal rate of weight loss is around 1-2lb (½-1kg) per week, although there is often a rapid loss in the beginning (mostly of water). A steady weight loss of around 4lb (2kg) per month is good.

Weight chart

Take a straight line across from your height (without shoes) and a line up from your weight (without clothes). Mark where the two lines meet.

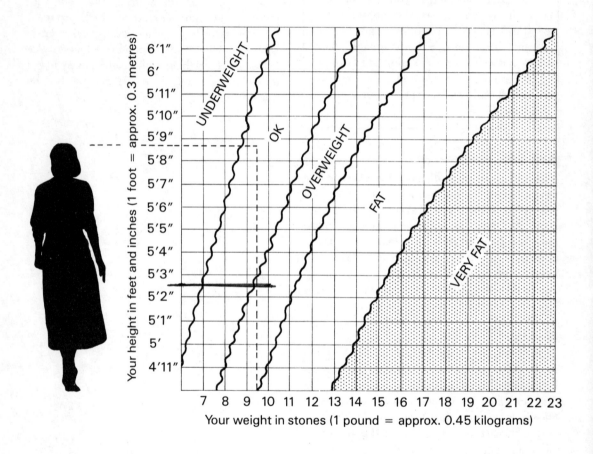

From Garrow JS (1981), *Treat Obesity Seriously*. Edinburgh: Churchill Livingstone.

Underweight Maybe you need to eat a bit more, but go for well-balanced nutritious foods and don't just fill up on fatty and sugary foods. If you are *very* underweight, see your doctor about it.

OK You're eating the right *quantity* of food but you need to be sure that you're getting a healthy *balance* in your diet.

Overweight You should try to lose weight.

Fat You need to lose weight.

Very fat You urgently need to lose weight. You would do well to see your doctor, who might refer you to a dietitian.

If you need to lose weight, aim to lose 1 or 2 lb (½-1kg) a week until you get down to the 'OK' range. Go for fibre-rich foods and cut down on fat, sugar and alcohol. You'll need to take regular exercise too.

Use the recipes in this book to help you follow the healthy eating guidelines. Each recipe has been given a calorie value to help you keep track of how much you are eating.

If you have insulin dependent diabetes, changing your diet may mean you have to inject less insulin. It is best to consult your doctor and dietitian before adopting a reduced calorie, and probably carbohydrate, diet.

What happens next? Often after getting your weight down successfully, it slowly starts to creep up again as you allow yourself more treats. Once you are satisfied with your weight, gradually include more variety, especially of the high fibre starchy foods. Start, for example, by having an extra slice of bread or an extra helping of potatoes and then slowly introduce more of the other foods you enjoy. Continue to step on the scales regularly so that you can keep your new weight in check.

Lastly, good luck — you *can* do it!

About carbohydrate

The amount of carbohydrate (CHO) or starchy foods eaten daily is an important consideration for people with diabetes. It is often felt that people with diabetes should cut down on starchy foods. This is not true. In the past, a low CHO diet was encouraged. However, it has since been shown that if around half your daily calorie intake comes from high-CHO, high-fibre foods, then your blood sugar level will improve. This is obviously better in the long term. The starchy foods recommended in the section Fibre on page 18 are the best types to choose. The soluble fibre they contain has the most favourable effect on blood glucose and may also help reduce blood cholesterol levels.

Latest developments

Many studies have been conducted in this field and you may hear rumours that this amount of CHO can make your control worse, instead of improving it. Don't worry! After an extensive review of all the research that has been published, the British Diabetic Association still

Introducing diabetes

feels that a high-CHO, low-fat diet is the most appropriate for people with diabetes, *provided the diet is high in soluble fibre*, particularly in its whole, unprocessed form. The Canadian, Australian, American and European Associations also encourage a high-CHO, high-fibre, low-fat diet.

What is a 'CHO exchange'?

All meals eaten by people with diabetes must contain some CHO. To help people with diabetes control their CHO intake and still enjoy varied and interesting meals, a system of 'exchanges' has been developed. An exchange refers to a particular amount of CHO. One apple and one orange each contain approximately 10g of CHO, and can thus be 'exchanged', or swapped, for one another.

CHO 'exchange lists' are used by some insulin dependent diabetics, but they can be impractical. Many people prefer to use ordinary household measures (cups, spoons and so on) to weighing food. It may be that general advice on the quantity of the diet and the best mix of foods

will eventually replace the CHO counting system. Placing so much emphasis on CHO is considered by many experts to be misleading as CHO is not the only nutrient that you need to adjust when you have diabetes. Far more important is the *whole diet:* the mix of foods that are eaten and when, how long they are cooked and whether they are puréed or eaten whole.

Exchange lists are, however, still very much in use. In Canada and America, in fact, up to nine food exchange lists may be used. The European Association for the Study of Diabetes, while currently recommending CHO exchange systems, acknowledges that better exchange lists should be developed. These lists should encourage the use of the more beneficial type of CHO, high-soluble fibre carbohydrates.

Each recipe in this book has been given a carefully calculated CHO value — this will be useful to you if your dietitian has prescribed a daily CHO allowance.

Use this book to ensure that you select the foods that are the most appropriate for good control of your diabetes and also for good health.

About the recipes

All the recipes in this book have been prepared in a healthy way. High-fibre, low-fat ingredients have been used and low-fat cooking methods have been chosen. Each recipe has been carefully tried and tested. The calorie and carbohydrate content of each recipe has been accurately calculated using up-to-date professional nutrition tables.

The ingredients used

Fat
- wherever possible, polyunsaturated and monounsaturated oils (try to use mono-unsaturated oils more often)
- low-fat spread (including polyunsaturated low-fat spread)
- lean meat and poultry or low-fat dairy products

Fibre
- lentils, beans, wholemeal pasta, brown rice, wholemeal flour, oats, dried fruit, fresh fruit and vegetables

Sugar
- small amounts of ordinary sugar in baking
- artificial sweeteners in desserts where sugar is not required.

Weights and measures

Quantities of ingredients have been given in both metric and imperial measurements. The metric measurements have been used for the calculations. Choose whichever system of measurement you prefer, but use either *all* metric or *all* imperial, otherwise you risk a poor result, especially with pastry, breads and cakes.

Recipe calculations

All calculations are based on raw ingredients, unless the word 'cooked' appears in the ingredient list.

Carbohydrate (CHO) calculations

The section About carbohydrate on page 33 explained why CHO is important in diabetes. Not all foods contain CHO. For example, many vegetables — such as lettuce, tomato, carrots and cabbage — and fruits — such as rhubarb, lemons, raspberries and gooseberries — have such small amounts of CHO that it does not make sense to count them (these are listed in Table 1, page 15). The same is true for flavourings such as stock and tomato purée. If a food contains less than 5g of CHO, it is considered negligible (referred to as 'neg.' in the recipes). The list below is of the vegetables that have been counted when making CHO calculations for the recipes in this book:

- baked beans
- pulses and beans, such as chick peas, split peas, lentils
- potatoes.

It is more practical to round up or down to the nearest 10g rather than to use the exact CHO value. For example, if a recipe has 23g of CHO per portion, this has been rounded down to 20g. This makes CHO counting much easier.

Calorie calculations

All foods provide calories, but in some cases the number of calories is so minute that it is not necessary to count them. In this book, seasonings, certain condiments (such as vinegar and lemon juice) and artificial sweeteners have not been calorie counted.

Although some vegetables (such as cabbage and carrots) are very low in calories, their calorie content has been included in the recipe calculations to make them as accurate as possible. However, on a day-to-day basis the calories from these vegetables need not be counted, so eat them freely — choose from the list in Table 1 on page 15.

As with CHO, the exact calorie content of the ingredients has been assessed. The total figure for the recipe has then been rounded up or down to the nearest 10 kcalories.

Adapting your own recipes for home baking

No one is suggesting that you should throw away all your favourite recipes and cookbooks just because you are now following a healthy eating plan. Instead, modify them by reducing the amount of saturated fat and sugar they contain and increasing the amount of fibre. You may find the following guidelines useful:

- if a recipe calls for white flour, try using wholemeal flour instead or half wholemeal and half white. This gives a lighter texture than wholemeal on its own for sponge cakes and so on
- replacing butter and ordinary margarine with low-fat spread can reduce the fat and calories by half, but some of these spreads do not work well in baking, so polyunsaturated margarines are a useful alternative. (Remember, however, that these margarines have exactly the same quantity of fat and calories as ordinary butter, although they do have the advantage of being high in polyunsaturated fat so using a polyunsaturated low-fat spread gives you the best of both worlds; look out, too, for new low-fat products designed especially for baking)

- in most cases, you can reduce the sugar content of a traditional recipe (such as for a Victoria sandwich) by half: proportions of up to 50g (2oz) of sugar to 225g (8oz) of flour give satisfactory results in rock cakes, scones, fruit loaves and so on and, on average, this yields between 2 and 5g of sugar per scone, which is the same as a couple of digestive biscuits
- remember that if you use sugar, it does add to the carbohydrate content of a recipe
- not everyone needs to count their calories and CHO and you are certainly not expected to own food composition tables such as those that have been used in the compiling of this book, but if you are on a CHO allowance, the table below may be of help.

Practical cooking tips

- Try baking cakes using less sugar than a traditional recipe demands. In some cases you can use only half the normal amount still concoct a mouthwatering treat. How about a Victoria Sandwich (see page 155) for a high-fibre, low-sugar accompaniment to afternoon tea?
- If making custard, use skimmed milk, custard powder and an artificial sweetener.
- Make your own jelly using low-calorie squash, unsweetened fruit juice and gelatine.
- Include beans, peas and lentils in recipes that contain meat. Replacing some of the meat with beans is cheaper and very nutritious.
- Use reduced or low-fat spread, preferably monounsaturated (if available) or polyunsaturated, for baking — try the Banana and Walnut Slices on page 158). Use non-stick cookware, too.
- Remove the skin from poultry and trim the fat off meat.
- Choose refreshing fruity desserts such as the Raspberry and Kiwi Whip on page 142, rather than rich stodgy puds.

Ingredients	CHO (in grams)
25g (1oz) flour (any kind)	20
25g (1oz) sugar (any kind)	30
Polyunsaturated margarine or low-fat spread	No carbohydrate content
Eggs	No carbohydrate content
185ml (⅓pt) of milk (any kind)	10
25g (1oz) dried fruit (any kind)	20
Up to 100g (4oz) nuts	Negligible carbohydrate content
Up to 50g (2oz) cocoa powder	Negligible carbohydrate content

- Reduce the amount of salt you use in cooking as we eat far more salt than we need. Flavour your food with lemon juice, herbs, spices or mustard instead for healthier, tastier food.
- Eat more oily fish, such as herring and mackerel, that are high in polyunsaturated fat and are still moist after grilling.
- Grill, bake, poach, steam or boil foods rather than frying them. Twenty-five g (1oz) of boiled potato provides about 20 kcalories — make this amount of potato into chips and the calories multiply three times!
- Choose oils that are high in monounsaturated fat (such as olive oil) or polyunsaturated fat (such as corn oil) and, even so, remember to use as little as possible. Also, remember that polyunsaturated oil becomes more saturated when it is reused, which makes it less desirable in your diet, but that monounsaturated oils are not altered when they are reused. So, when frying, choose a monounsaturated oil if you are planning to reuse it.
- Use low-fat dairy products in recipes, such as skimmed or semi-skimmed milk, reduced-fat cheeses and low-fat yogurt. Low-fat cream cheese and low-fat yogurt make good substitutes for cream. How about making the Yogurt Gooseberry Fool on page 142?
- Beans don't necessarily need to be the dried variety, which require soaking. Tinned beans are just as healthy and can be used straight away.
- Keep the skins on potatoes. This doesn't mean having potatoes baked in their jackets day in, day out — roasted, scalloped, sautéd or boiled potatoes can all be cooked with their skins on and you benefit from the extra fibre.
- Brown rice contains more fibre than white. Try it sometime. (Remember, though, that you need more water for brown rice and it takes longer to cook.)
- Use half wholemeal and half white flour for baking — you don't need to use wholemeal on its own, which can be quite dry in some baked goods. Simply choose what you and your family find tastes good.

The Recipes

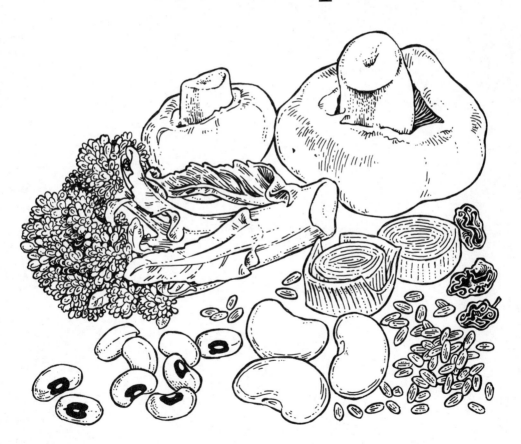

Soups and starters

An enticing starter often paves the way for good things to come. Starters should complement the main course. It's best to serve small portions and to present them attractively with eye-catching garnishes.

Cold starters can be prepared in advance, enabling you to deal with other parts of the meal or to talk with your guests. Serve pâtés or dips with raw, fresh vegetables such as carrots, celery and cauliflower florets to help add fibre to a meal simply.

Delicious, home-made soup is always welcoming on a cold winter's day. They are extremely nourishing and can be transformed into a light main meal if served with wholegrain granary rolls or bread. The use of vegetables and pulses in the soups helps to increase the fibre — and taste — content.

Taramasalata

Serves 8-10

8 small slices wholemeal bread
175g (6 oz) fresh smoked cod roe, skinned
juice of 1-2 lemons
1 slice onion
1 clove garlic, crushed
50ml (2 fl oz) oil
olives, to garnish

Soak the bread in water for 10 minutes. Squeeze it gently then put it in a food processor or blender. Add the roe, lemon juice, onion and garlic. Blend for 2 minutes until well mixed. Slowly add the oil while the blender is running. Blend for 1-2 minutes.

COOK'S TIP
If a milder taste is preferred, add a little more bread and oil.
If it is too stiff, add 1-2 teaspoons water. The consistency should be neither
runny nor too stiff, but rather, a spreadable consistency.
Serve on a platter and garnish with olives.

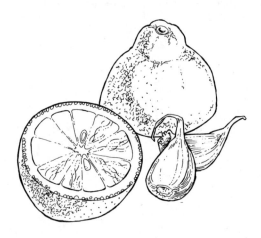

Minestrone Soup

Serves 6-8

2 tbs olive oil
75g (3 oz) rindless streaky bacon, chopped
1 onion, chopped
1 clove garlic, crushed
3 stalks celery, chopped
2 small carrots, finely chopped
1 courgette, chopped
25g (1 oz) small pasta shells, bows or similar
salt and freshly ground black pepper
1 tsp dried oregano or basil
1 tbs tomato purée
1.1l (2 pt) chicken stock
225-g (1×8-oz) tin red kidney beans, drained and refreshed
under cold running water
a little grated Parmesan cheese

Heat the oil in a large saucepan. Add the bacon, onion and garlic and fry until the bacon is crisp. Stir in the remaining vegetables (except the kidney beans) and pasta. Add seasonings, tomato purée and stock. Bring to boil, stirring constantly. Reduce the heat, cover and simmer for 20-25 minutes, stirring occasionally. Add the kidney beans and simmer for a further 10 minutes or until all the vegetables are tender. Adjust the seasoning to taste before serving and sprinkle with the Parmesan cheese.

Tomato Soup

Serves 4

1 tbs corn or sunflower oil
1 medium-sized onion, peeled and chopped
2 rashers streaky bacon, rinds removed and chopped
1 tbs flour
450g (1 lb) fresh tomatoes, halved and deseeded
550ml (1 pt) chicken stock
salt and freshly ground black pepper
pinch dried basil
lemon juice to taste
1 tsp intense sweetener

Heat the oil in a pan, add the onion and bacon and cook for 5 minutes. Stir in the flour and cook for 1 minute, stirring constantly. Add the tomatoes and gradually stir in the stock. Bring to the boil, then reduce the heat and add the seasonings. Simmer for 20 minutes.

Remove the pan from the heat and rub the soup through a sieve. Adjust the seasoning to taste, add lemon juice and sweetener then serve.

Lentil Soup

Serves 4

2 onions, peeled and chopped
3 carrots, chopped
100g (4 oz) lentils
1.1l (2 pt) ham stock
freshly ground black pepper
fresh parsley, to garnish

Put the onions, carrots, lentils and stock in a pan. Bring to the boil, then cover and simmer for 40-45 minutes, stirring occasionally.

Either liquidize the soup or rub it through a sieve. Adjust the seasoning to taste, then serve, garnished with parsley.

Watercress and Onion Soup

CHO neg
Kcals 90

Serves 4

1 bunch watercress, washed and roughly chopped
2 onions, peeled and chopped
550ml (1 pt) vegetable stock
a little grated nutmeg
salt and freshly ground black pepper
a few watercress leaves to garnish

Put the watercress and onions in a pan. Add the stock and seasonings. Bring to the boil, cover and simmer for 20 minutes. Leave to cool slightly, then pour the soup into a blender or liquidizer and blend until smooth. Return the soup to the pan and reheat. Adjust the seasoning to taste. Serve garnished with the watercress.

Turkey or Chicken Broth

CHO neg
Kcals 200

Serves 4

1 chicken or turkey carcass and any leftover meat diced
3 carrots, peeled and diced
2 leeks, thinly sliced
2 tbs rice
1 bay leaf
salt and freshly ground black pepper

Put the carcass in a large pan and cover with water. Add the remaining ingredients and bring to the boil. Reduce the heat and simmer for 2 hours, skimming any froth and fat with a spoon when necessary. Add more water if the liquid in the pan becomes low.

To serve, remove the carcass from the pan. Skim the soup well to remove any remaining fat and adjust the seasoning to taste, then serve.

Soups and starters

Smoked Mackerel Pâté

CHO neg
Kcals 560

Serves 4

225g (8 oz) smoked mackerel fillets
100g (4 oz) skimmed milk soft cheese
lemon juice to taste
salt and freshly ground black pepper

Flake the fish into a bowl. Add the soft cheese and lemon juice and season to taste. Mix the ingredients together well by hand or process in a liquidizer or blender. Put the pâté into a serving dish and chill until needed. Will keep in refrigerator for up to 48 hours.

Chicken Liver Pâté

CHO neg
Kcals 430

Serves 4

25g (1 oz) low-fat spread
1 medium onion, finely chopped
225g (8 oz) chicken livers
1 tsp grated nutmeg
salt and freshly ground black pepper
1 slice lemon

Put the low-fat spread in a pan and lightly sauté the onion for 1 minute. Add the chicken livers and seasonings. Continue cooking for 5-6 minutes, stirring occasionally. Leave them to cool, then liquidize or blend until smooth. Put the pâté into the serving dish and smooth the top. Put the lemon slice on top. Chill until needed. Will keep in the refrigerator for up to 48 hours.

Stuffed Pears

Serves 4

2 dessert pears, cut in half, core removed and sprinkled with lemon juice
100g (4 oz) cottage cheese
25g (1 oz) walnuts, chopped
1 tbs raisins
few drops Worcestershire sauce
salt and freshly ground black pepper
lettuce and tomato or lemon slices to garnish

Put the pear halves on a lettuce leaf. Put to one side. Meanwhile, put the remaining ingredients in a bowl and mix them together well. Pile the mixture into the pear halves and garnish with the tomato or lemon slices, then serve immediately.

Guacamole

Serves 4-6

2 ripe avocados, about 100g (4 oz) each
juice of 1 lemon
1 small onion, peeled and finely chopped
1 clove garlic, crushed
225g (½ lb) tomatoes, skinned, de-seeded and finely chopped
dash of Tabasco sauce
fresh parsley, chopped to garnish

Scoop the flesh out from the avocados into a bowl. Mash the lemon juice into the flesh. Add the remaining ingredients and blend well until the mixture is quite smooth. Chill until needed, then transfer it to a serving dish and sprinkle the parsley over it.

Slimmer's Salad

Serves 4-6

450g (1 lb) cottage cheese
1×150-g (1×5-fl oz) carton low-fat natural yogurt
2 tbs fresh chives, chopped
½ cucumber, diced
1 red pepper, deseeded and diced
½ onion, grated
salt and freshly ground black pepper
a few lettuce leaves, shredded, to garnish

Combine the cottage cheese with the yogurt, chives, cucumber, and pepper. Season to taste with the onion, salt and pepper and toss together well. Serve on a bed of the lettuce.

Mediterranean-style Mackerel

Serves 4

2 tbs olive oil
1 onion, chopped
1 clove garlic, crushed
1 medium aubergine, cut into small cubes
2 tomatoes, chopped
1 tsp oregano
1 mackerel, filleted
salt and freshly ground black pepper

Heat the oil in a pan and sauté the onions and garlic until tender. Add the aubergine and cook for 5 minutes. Add the tomatoes, seasonings and fish and simmer for 20 minutes. Lift out the fish and put it on a serving dish. Serve it topped with the vegetables.

Meat and poultry

Family meals are often quite a challenge — making food that satisfies everybody's likes and dislikes and doesn't break the budget. We've put together a selection of some family favourites and adapted them so that they are healthier without sacrificing taste.

Inventive use of nourishing economical foods like the cheaper cuts of meat and fish, fresh vegetables in season and dairy products all help to produce delicious inexpensive meals.

Casseroles and stews are tasty, easy to make and to reheat if your family needs to have staggered mealtimes.

Another good idea is to add beans and other pulses to meat dishes. Not only does this increase the fibre but it makes the meat go further.

Stuffed Peppers and Tomatoes

CHO 80g
Kcals 1570

Serves 4

4 green peppers
4 large tomatoes
2 tbs tomato purée diluted in 150ml (¼ pt) hot water
1 tbs corn or sunflower oil

Stuffing
225g (8 oz) lean, minced beef or lamb
1 large onion, chopped
150ml (¼ pt) hot water
2 tbs fresh parsley, finely chopped
salt and freshly ground black pepper
50g (2 oz) brown rice, cooked
50g (2 oz) pine kernels
50g (2 oz) sultanas

Cut a slice off the top of each pepper and tomato and reserve them. Deseed the peppers. Scoop out most of the tomato flesh, chop it and reserve it for the stuffing.

To make the stuffing, cook the meat and onions in a pan until they brown. Add the hot water, the reserved tomato flesh and seasoning ingredients. Mix well and cook for 15 minutes. Add the remaining ingredients, mix well and cook for 3 minutes. Arrange the tomatoes and peppers upright in a baking dish. Fill them with the stuffing, leaving a little room for it to expand and replace the reserved tops.

Pour the tomato purée mixture over them and cook at 375°F/190°C (Gas Mark 5) for 1 hour and 10 minutes, basting them occasionally. If all the liquid evaporates, add a few tablespoons of water.

Stuffed Vine Leaves

Serves 4-6

1 packet of fresh vine leaves
2 cloves garlic, crushed
1 × 400-g (14-oz) tin chopped tomatoes
salt and freshly ground black pepper
275ml (½ pt) hot water

Stuffing
100g (4 oz) brown rice, washed and drained
225g (8 oz) minced lamb or beef
1 egg, beaten
1 large onion, finely sliced
50g (2 oz) pine kernels
½ tsp cinnamon (optional)
3 tbs fresh parsley, chopped

Follow the instructions for preparing the leaves on the packet. Mix all the stuffing ingredients together well, then put a heaped teaspoon of the stuffing at the centre of each leaf. Fold the side edges inwards and then the top part, then roll tightly to the bottom of the leaf. Mix the garlic, tomatoes and salt and pepper together. Pack the rolls tightly together in circles in a saucepan, with the folded edge downwards, layering them with the tomato mixture. Put an inverted small heat-proof plate on top (to keep them in place and prevent them unrolling) and pour in the hot water, which should come up to just under the surface. Cover and cook gently for 1 hour. Serve hot.

Meat and poultry

Broccoli in Ham and Cheese Sauce

CHO 30g
Kcals 540

Serves 2

225g (8 oz) broccoli, cut into even-sized pieces
25g (1 oz) low-fat spread
25g (1 oz) wholemeal flour
275ml (½ pt) skimmed milk
50g (2 oz) reduced-fat cheddar cheese, grated
50g (2 oz) lean ham, finely chopped
1 tsp wholegrain mustard
salt and freshly ground black pepper

Cook the broccoli until just tender but still crisp. Meanwhile, make the sauce.

Melt the low-fat spread over a low heat, add the flour and stir over the heat for 1 minute. Gradually add the milk, stirring, and bring to the boil. Reduce the heat and simmer for about 3 minutes. Reserve a tablespoon of the cheese and stir the remainder into the sauce. Stir in the ham, mustard and seasoning.

Arrange the broccoli in an ovenproof dish, pour the cheese sauce over it and sprinkle the reserved cheese over the top. Grill until the grated cheese melts and turns golden brown. Serve immediately.

Pork Stir-fry

Serves 4

1 tbs olive or sunflower oil
350g (12 oz) lean pork tenderloin fillet, cut into thin strips
2.5-cm (1-in) piece root ginger, peeled and finely chopped
1 carrot, peeled and diced
1 onion, peeled and finely chopped
2 small courgettes, washed and sliced
100g (4 oz) baby sweetcorn
225g (8 oz) beansprouts
2 tbs dry sherry
2 tbs light soy sauce
freshly ground black pepper

Heat the oil in a wok or large frying pan. Add the pork, ginger and onion and stir-fry for 5 to 10 minutes or until the pork is cooked. Add the carrot, onion, courgettes and corn and stir-fry for 5 to 10 minutes. Stir in the beansprouts, sherry and soy sauce. Mix well and stir-fry for 1 minute. Season to taste with freshly ground black pepper and serve immediately.

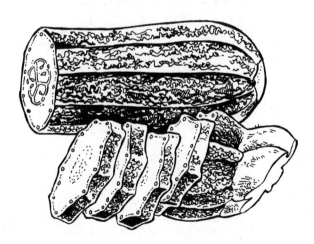

Meat and poultry

Sweet-and-sour Chicken

CHO 30g
Kcals 760

Serves 4

1 tbs olive or sunflower oil
3 boneless chicken breasts, skin removed, diced
1 onion, sliced
1 green pepper, deseeded and chopped
1 red pepper, deseeded and chopped
225-g (1×8-oz) tin tomatoes
225-g (1×8-oz) tin pineapple pieces in natural juice
1 tbs vinegar
1 tbs soy sauce
about 150ml (¼ pt) water
salt and freshly ground black pepper

Heat the oil and lightly fry the chicken and onion for 5 minutes. Add the remaining ingredients. Bring to the boil, stirring, cover and simmer for 20-30 minutes or until the chicken is tender, adding a little more water if it starts to get a bit dry.

Stir-fried Chicken with Cashews

CHO 30g
Kcals 1090

Serves 4

4 boneless, skinless chicken breasts, cut into even-sized pieces
2.5-cm (1-in) piece root ginger, peeled and chopped
2-3 cloves garlic, crushed
1-2 tsp cornflour
1 tbs dry sherry
1 tbs light soy sauce
150ml (¼ pt) chicken stock
1 tbs olive or sunflower oil
50g (2 oz) unsalted cashew nuts
salt and freshly ground black pepper

Put the chicken, ginger and garlic in a bowl and leave to stand. Meanwhile, mix the cornflower with the sherry, soy sauce and chicken stock. Heat the oil in a large frying pan or wok. Add the nuts and stir-fry until they are lightly browned. Remove them, then add the chicken, ginger and garlic and stir-fry until the chicken is cooked and tender. Add the sherry, soy sauce and stock mixture and stir until the liquid has thickened. If the sauce becomes too thick, add a little water. Season to taste with salt and freshly ground black pepper. Add the cashew nuts, mix them in well, heat it through, then serve immediately.

Lemon and Herb Baked Chicken

CHO neg
Kcals 370

Serves 2

2 skinless, boned chicken breasts
juice of half a lemon
2 tsp olive or sunflower oil
1 clove garlic, crushed
freshly ground black pepper
pinch of mixed herbs

Score the chicken breasts with a sharp knife and lay them in an ovenproof dish. In a small bowl, mix the lemon juice, oil, garlic, pepper and herbs. Spoon the mixture over the chicken, leave to marinate for 30 minutes. Then bake at 375°F/190°C (Gas Mark 5) for 30 minutes, until the chicken is cooked.

Greek-style Lamb Kebabs

CHO neg
Kcals 1820

Serves 4-6

2 tbs corn or sunflower oil
juice of ½ a lemon
1-2 cloves of garlic, crushed
675g (1½ lb) boned leg of lamb, cut into cubes
salt
cayenne pepper

Beat the oil, lemon juice and garlic together and let the meat marinate in it for 4 hours, covered in a refrigerator, basting the meat occasionally. Thread the meat onto skewers and grill for 8-10 minutes, turning the skewers to brown the meat on all sides. Brush the kebabs with the marinade once or twice. Allow an extra 5 minutes if cooking on a barbecue. Season with salt and cayenne pepper to taste and serve immediately.

Minced Beef Cobbler

CHO 80g
Kcals 1140

Serves 4

450g (1 lb) extra lean minced beef
1 onion, peeled and chopped
2 carrots, peeled and diced
227-g (1×8-oz) tin tomatoes
about 150ml (¼ pt) beef stock
salt and freshly ground black pepper

Cobbler
100g (4 oz) fine self-raising wholemeal flour
1 tsp baking powder
pinch salt
25g (1 oz) low-fat spread
150ml (¼ pt) skimmed milk

Sauté the mince, onion and carrots in a saucepan until the mince is all lightly browned. Add the tomatoes and stock and simmer for 30 minutes, stirring occasionally. Season to taste with salt and freshly ground black pepper.

Meanwhile, rub the fat into the flour, baking powder and salt until the mixture resembles fine breadcrumbs, then stir in enough milk to form a soft dough. Roll it out on a lightly floured surface until it is 1cm (½ in) thick and, using a 5-cm (2-in) cutter, cut out circles.

Pour the mince mixture into an ovenproof dish and place the dough 'cobbles' around the edge, overlapping them. Brush them with the remaining milk and bake at 400°F/200°C (Gas Mark 6) for 10-12 minutes, until the cobbler has risen and turned golden brown. Serve immediately, giving everyone a serving of the cobbler with their savoury mince.

Beefburger Surprise

CHO neg
Kcals 700

Serves 4

450g (1 lb) extra lean minced beef
1 onion, peeled and finely chopped
salt and freshly ground black pepper
50g (2 oz) reduced-fat cheddar cheese

Put the mince, onion and seasonings into a bowl and mix them together well. Divide the mixture in half and shape each into an 18-cm (7-in) round. Sprinkle the cheese evenly over one round to within 1 cm (½ in) of the edges. Cover the cheese layer with the second round and pinch the edges together firmly, sealing the filling inside.

Cook the burger under the grill for approximately 6-8 minutes each side, or until cooked through. Cut it into quarters and serve.

Meat and poultry

Cottage Pie

CHO 60g
Kcals 900

Serves 4-6

450g (1 lb) extra lean minced beef
1 onion, peeled and chopped
2 carrots, peeled and finely chopped
227-g (1×8-oz) tin tomatoes
1 tbs tomato purée
about 150ml (¼ pt) beef stock
salt and freshly ground black pepper
350g (12 oz) potatoes, peeled, boiled and mashed

Sauté the minced beef, onions and carrots until the meat is all just brown, stirring occasionally. Stir in the tomatoes, tomato purée and stock. Season to taste with salt and freshly ground black pepper, cover and simmer for 30 minutes.

Spoon the mixture into an ovenproof dish and spread the mashed potato over the meat.

Decorate the surface of the potato by drawing wavy lines on it with a fork.

Bake the pie in the oven at 375°F/190°C (Gas Mark 5) for 30-35 minutes. If liked, place the pie under the grill just before serving to crispen the potato topping.

Macaroni Mince

CHO 40g
Kcals 890

Serves 4

450g (1 lb) extra lean minced beef
2 medium onions, finely chopped
1 clove garlic, crushed
1 medium carrot, finely diced
227-g (1×8-oz) tin tomatoes
salt and freshly ground black pepper
pinch of mixed herbs
about 150ml (¼ pt) beef stock
50g (2 oz) wholewheat macaroni, cooked
25g (1 oz) half-fat hard cheese, grated

Put the mince, onion, garlic and carrot in a pan and fry gently until all the mince has browned, stirring occasionally. Stir in the remaining ingredients and seasonings except the macaroni and cheese, bring to the boil and simmer for 20 minutes.

Once cooked, pour half the mince mixture into an ovenproof dish, then add the macaroni in a layer. Put the remaining mince over the macaroni and top with the grated cheese. Brown the cheese under the grill, then serve hot.

Spaghetti Bolognese

CHO neg
Kcals 560

+ Spaghetti counts

Serves 4

350g (12 oz) extra lean minced beef
1 onion, finely chopped
1 clove garlic, crushed
2 carrots, finely chopped
2 sticks celery, thinly sliced
100g (4 oz) mushrooms, sliced
400-g (1×14-oz) tin tomatoes, chopped, with juice
1 tbs tomato purée
150ml (¼ pt) beef stock
½ tsp basil
½ tsp oregano
salt and freshly ground black pepper

Brown the minced beef in a large pan without added fat for 5 minutes. Drain off any excess fat, then add the onion, garlic, carrot, celery and mushrooms and stir well. Add the remaining ingredients and season to taste with salt and freshly ground black pepper. Bring to boil and simmer gently for 30-40 minutes, stirring occasionally. While the Bolognese sauce is cooking, bring a large pan of salted water to the boil and cook the spaghetti. When the spaghetti is *al dente* and the Bolognese sauce is ready, drain the spaghetti and either add it to the sauce and mix well together or serve a nest of spaghetti on each plate, topped with the Bolognese sauce. **Note** Remember to take into account the CHO values of any spaghetti. 45g cooked weight of wholemeal spaghetti = 10g CHO.

Meat and poultry

Moussaka

Serves 4-6

1 large aubergine (about 275g/10 oz), sliced and sprinkled with 1 tsp salt
2 tbs corn or sunflower oil
450g (1 lb) extra lean minced lamb
1 large onion, chopped
1 clove garlic, crushed
1 tsp cinnamon
2 tbs fresh parsley, chopped
salt and freshly ground black pepper
3 tbs tomato purée
340g (12 oz) potatoes, parboiled and thinly sliced

White sauce
25g (1 oz) low-fat spread
25g (1 oz) flour
275ml (½ pt) skimmed milk
salt and freshly ground black pepper
pinch of ground nutmeg
1 egg yolk

Once the aubergines have rendered their bitter juices, pat them dry with absorbent kitchen paper. Heat the oil in a large frying pan and fry the aubergine slices until they are golden brown on both sides. Drain them on absorbent kitchen paper. Meanwhile, sauté the lamb, onion and garlic until all the meat is brown. Add the cinnamon, parsley, salt and pepper to taste, tomato purée and a little water to moisten.

In a large, ovenproof casserole, put alternate layers of meat and aubergines starting and ending with a meat layer. Put a layer of the potatoes over the top.

Make the white sauce and allow it to cool slightly before mixing in the egg yolk. Spoon the sauce over the potatoes in the dish and bake at 375°F/190°C (Gas Mark 5) for 25-30 minutes or until the top is golden brown.

Navarin of Lamb

Serves 4

1 tbs corn or sunflower oil
1 large onion, chopped
1 clove garlic, crushed
4 chump chops, trimmed of fat
1 tbs flour
2 carrots, sliced
1 small swede (about 225g/½ lb), peeled and chopped
1 tbs tomato purée
400-g (1×14-oz) tin chopped tomatoes
1 bouquet garni
freshly ground black pepper
fresh parsley, chopped, to garnish

Heat the oil in a flameproof casserole. Add the onion and garlic and fry for 5 minutes.

Meanwhile, coat the lamb chops in the flour. Add them to the casserole and brown them quickly on both sides. Add the carrots, swede, tomato purée and tomatoes and bring to the boil.

Add the seasonings. Cover with a lid and transfer to oven and cook at 325°F/170°C (Gas Mark 3) for 1-2 hours, until the meat is tender. Adjust the seasoning to taste and sprinkle the chopped parsley over before serving.

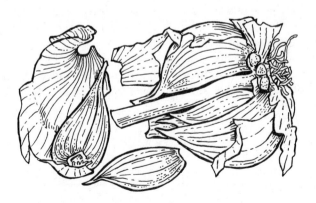

Beef Stew and Dumplings

CHO 100g
Kcals 2430

Serves 4

2 tbs corn or sunflower oil
675g (1½ lb) braising steak, trimmed and cut into cubes
3 sticks celery, sliced
3 small carrots, peeled and sliced
1 small swede (about 100g/4 oz), peeled and cubed
2 onions, peeled and chopped
2 tbs flour
2 tbs tomato purée
550ml (1 pt) beef stock
2 bay leaves
freshly ground black pepper

Dumpling mixture
100g (4 oz) self-raising wholemeal flour
50g (2 oz) vegetable suet
pinch salt
1 tbs parsley, chopped
sufficient water to bind

Heat the oil in a large, flameproof casserole. Add the meat and fry until it has browned to seal in the flavour (about 5 minutes). Add all the prepared vegetables and fry for 3 minutes. Stir in the flour and cook for 1 minute, stirring. Stir in the tomato purée, stock, bay leaves and seasoning and bring to the boil. Cover with the lid and bake at 350°F/180°C (Gas Mark 4) for 1-2 hours, until the meat is tender.

To make the dumplings, sift the flour into a bowl and stir in the suet, seasoning and parsley. Mix to a firm (not sticky) dough with water (about 5 tbs). Form into 8 dumplings and put them on top of the meat in the casserole for the last 20 minutes or so until the dumplings are light and fluffy (do not remove the lid during this 20 minutes).

Carbonade of Beef

CHO 10g
Kcals 1640

Serves 4

2 tbs corn or sunflower oil
675g (1½ lb) chuck steak, cut into cubes
1 onion, peeled and chopped
4 celery stalks, chopped
2 carrots, sliced
1 tbs flour
salt and freshly ground black pepper
1 tsp vinegar
1 bouquet garni
275ml (½ pt) stout
fresh parsley, chopped, to garnish

Heat the oil in a flameproof casserole, then add the cubes of meat and brown them quickly on all sides. Add the vegetables and cook for 5 minutes. Stir in flour, seasonings, vinegar, bouquet garni and stout. Cover the casserole and bake at 325°F/170°C (Gas Mark 3) for 1-2 hours, or until the meat is tender. Stir a little water into the casserole if it becomes dry during the cooking time. Discard the bouquet garni and adjust the seasoning to taste just before serving.

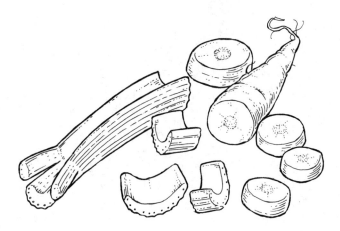

Meat and poultry

Barbecued Pork Chops

CHO neg
Kcals 430

Serves 2

2 lean pork chops or pork steaks

Barbecue sauce
1 tbs chilli sauce
1 tbs Worcestershire sauce
1 tbs vinegar
1 tbs tomato ketchup
1 tsp light soy sauce
1 clove garlic, crushed

Mix the barbecue sauce ingredients together. Put the chops or steaks in a casserole dish and bake at 375°F/190°C (Gas Mark 5) for approximately 10-15 minutes or until the chops are browned. Pour off any fat. Pour the sauce over them and recover. Bake for 25-30 more minutes, basting them occasionally. Arrange them on a serving dish and spoon the sauce over them.

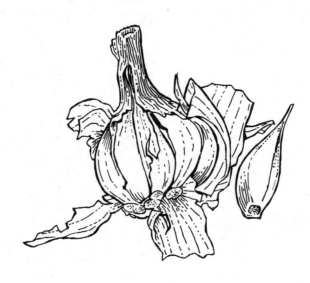

Fish

More people are eating more fish, which is good as it is a healthy, nutritious food. There are two main types of fish: the oily ones — such as mackerel — and white fish — such as cod, haddock and so on. The oils in oily fish are excellent sources of vitamins A and D and are also thought to protect the body against heart disease.

With the recipes in this chapter for both white and oily fish, you can cook up a tempting feast that will also benefit your general well-being.

Tuna Sauce

CHO neg
Kcals 420

Serves 3-4

1 tbs olive oil
2 cloves garlic, crushed
2-3 sticks celery, chopped
1 bay leaf
pinch oregano
salt and freshly ground black pepper
200-g (1×7-oz) tin tuna fish in brine, drained and flaked
400-g (1×14-oz) tin tomatoes
3 tbs tomato purée

Heat the oil in a pan and fry the garlic and celery. Add the herbs and seasoning to taste with salt and freshly ground black pepper. Stir in the tuna fish, tomatoes and tomato purée. Bring to the boil and simmer gently for 20-30 minutes.

Meanwhile cook the pasta in plenty of boiling salted water. Serve the tuna sauce as soon as it is ready on a bed of *al dente* pasta.

Note Remember to take into account the CHO values of any spaghetti: 45g cooked weight of wholemeal spaghetti = 10g CHO.

Baked Fish

CHO 10g
Kcals 850

Serves 4

4 cod steaks
3 tbs olive or sunflower oil
2 cloves garlic, finely sliced
4 tbs fresh parsley, finely chopped
450g (1 lb) tomatoes, deseeded and finely chopped
salt and freshly ground black pepper
2 tbs wholemeal breadcrumbs, toasted

Arrange the fish in a lightly oiled baking dish. Meanwhile, lightly beat together all other ingredients, apart from the breadcrumbs. Spread some of the mixture over each slice of fish, sprinkle with the breadcrumbs and bake at 375°F/190°C (Gas Mark 5) for 30-40 minutes, basting occasionally, until crisp on top.

COOK'S TIP
This dish is absolutely delicious served with boiled new potatoes and a green salad.

Smoked Haddock Plait

CHO 100g
Kcals 1310

Serves 4-6

25g (1 oz) low-fat spread
1 onion, peeled and chopped
25g (1 oz) flour
275ml (½ pt) skimmed milk
salt and freshly ground black pepper
1 tbs lemon juice
225g (8 oz) smoked haddock, cooked and flaked
50g (2 oz) sweetcorn
215g (7 oz) wholemeal puff pastry
1 hard-boiled egg, sliced
a little beaten egg to glaze

Heat the low-fat spread in a pan and sauté the onion. Add the flour and milk and stir continuously, until the sauce has thickened. Season to taste with salt and freshly ground black pepper. Add the lemon juice, fish and sweetcorn.

Roll the pastry out into an oblong shape 20 by 30 cm (8 by 12 in) and spoon the filling down the centre third of the pastry, layering it with the eggs.

Cut the pastry diagonally at 2-cm (1-in) intervals down each side of the oblong. Fold down the top and take one strip from each side of the pastry and cross them over the fish. Continue in this way to form a plait. Brush with the beaten egg and bake at 400°F/200°C (Gas Mark 6) for approximately 25 minutes, or until the pastry is golden brown.

Fish

Prawn and Cashew Nut Curry

CHO 20g
Kcals 930

Serves 4

1 tbs corn or sunflower oil
1 large onion, peeled and chopped
1-2 cloves garlic, crushed
1.5-cm (½-in) piece fresh root ginger, peeled and finely chopped
2 tsp ground coriander
2 tsp paprika
2 tsp ground cumin
400-g (1×14-oz) tin chopped tomatoes
350g (12 oz) frozen prawns, thawed
50g (2 oz) unsalted cashew nuts, lightly toasted and chopped
150-g (1×5-fl oz) carton low-fat natural yogurt
salt and freshly ground black pepper

Heat the oil in a pan and gently fry the onion, garlic and ginger. Add the spices and fry for about a minute. Add the chopped tomatoes, prawns and nuts and stir together well. Stir in the yogurt and seasonings and heat gently for about 5 minutes. Serve immediately.

Note Remember to take into account the CHO values of any rice — 3 tbs / 3×15ml spoonfuls = 10g CHO.

Paprika Fish

Serves 4

1 tbs corn or sunflower oil
2 onions, peeled and sliced
2 medium-size potatoes, peeled and cut into 2-cm (¾-in) dice
1 green pepper, deseeded and cut into strips
1 red pepper, deseeded and cut into strips
1-2 tbs paprika
salt and freshly ground black pepper
about 210ml (7 fl oz) water
675g (1½ lb) haddock fillet, cut into strips

Heat the oil in a pan, add the onion and potato and cook over a low heat, stirring frequently, for 5 minutes. Add the peppers and paprika and season with salt and freshly ground black pepper. Mix in the water and simmer over a low heat for approximately 20 minutes until the vegetables are tender.

Add the fish and simmer for a further 5-6 minutes until the fish is just cooked. Serve immediately.

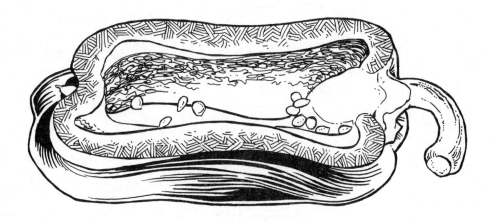

Fish-stuffed Baked Potatoes

Serves 4

4 medium-sized baking potatoes, washed
225g (8 oz) white fish
100g (4 oz) skimmed-milk cheese
1 clove garlic, crushed
1 tbs fresh chives, finely chopped
salt and freshly ground black pepper

Bake the potatoes at 400°F/200°C (Gas Mark 6) for approximately 1 hour or until potatoes are tender.

Meanwhile, steam the fish for about 6 minutes until just tender and flake it into a bowl, removing any bones and skin. When the potatoes are cooked, cut a slice off the top of each potato and scoop out the flesh into a bowl. Mash it with the cheese and garlic. Fold in the fish and chives and season to taste with salt and freshly ground black pepper. Fill each potato shell with the mixture and bake them at 350°F/180°C (Gas Mark 4) for 10-15 minutes or until the filling has heated through. Serve immediately.

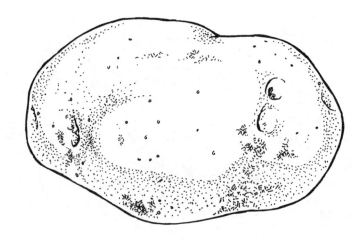

Prawn and Rice Salad

CHO 140g
Kcals 1210

Serves 4-6

175g (6 oz) brown rice, cooked
225g (8 oz) frozen prawns, defrosted
4 spring onions, finely chopped
1 green pepper, deseeded and chopped
2 tomatoes, chopped
salt and freshly ground black pepper
fresh parsley, chopped, to garnish

Dressing
3 tbs olive oil
1 tbs lemon juice
pinch mixed herbs

Put the rice in a bowl. Mix the dressing ingredients in a screw-top jar and pour it over the rice. Add the prawns, spring onion, pepper, tomatoes and seasoning and mix them together well. Serve garnished with the parsley.

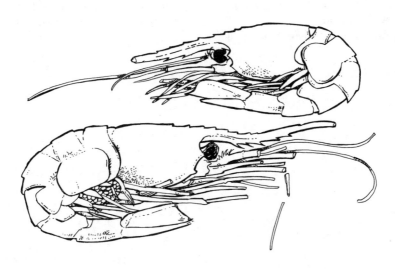

Cod and Avocado Salad

Serves 4

350g (12 oz) cod fillet
6 peppercorns
1 bay leaf
1 tbs white wine vinegar
7.5-cm (3-in) piece cucumber, sliced
2 tomatoes, sliced
1 avocado (about 175g/6 oz), peeled, stoned and chopped

Dressing
2 tbs lemon juice
2 tbs olive oil
1 tsp Dijon mustard
2 tbs fresh parsley, chopped
salt and freshly ground black pepper

Put the cod, peppercorns, bay leaf and vinegar in a pan with a little water. Cover and poach for 10-15 minutes until the fish is tender. Remove it carefully and leave it to cool.

Mix the fish lightly with the cucumber, tomato and avocado. Put the dressing ingredients in a screw-top jar and shake it well to mix. Pour the dressing over the salad and toss everything together lightly. Serve immediately.

Mackerel with Lime

CHO neg
Kcals 2060

Serves 4

4 mackerel (each about 225g/8 oz), gutted and filleted
2 limes, peeled and sliced
bunch spring onions, chopped
salt and freshly ground black pepper
150ml (¼ pt) dry cider
2 bay leaves

Put the mackerel in a lightly greased baking dish. Arrange the lime slices and spring onions down the middle of each fish and season with salt and freshly ground black pepper. Close each fish up and secure with wooden cocktail sticks. Pour the cider over them and add the bay leaves. Cover and cook at 350°F/180°C (Gas Mark 4) for 30-40 minutes or until tender. Serve hot.

Kedgeree

CHO 70g
Kcals 750

Serves 4

450g (1 lb) smoked haddock
150ml (¼ pt) skimmed milk
75g (3 oz) brown rice, cooked
1 size 3 egg, hard-boiled
100g (4 oz) frozen peas, cooked
salt and freshly ground black pepper
fresh parsley, chopped, to garnish

Poach the fish in the milk for 10-12 minutes or until tender. Drain, reserving the liquor. Remove any skin from the fish and flake the flesh. Add the fish and rice to a pan. Stir in the egg, and a little of the fish liquor. Season to taste with salt and freshly ground black pepper, then cook gently over a low heat until heated through. Serve immediately, garnished with the parsley.

Fish Salad Platter

Serves 4

225g (8 oz) cod fillet, cooked and flaked
2 tbs low-calorie French dressing
2 tsp lemon juice
1 × 200-g (7-oz) tin tuna in brine, drained
2 × size 3 eggs, hard-boiled and quartered
salt and freshly ground black pepper
1 lettuce, washed
3 tomatoes, sliced
1 green pepper, deseeded and sliced
6 black olives, halved, to garnish

Put the cod in a bowl. Add the French dressing and lemon juice. Add the tuna and eggs. Toss lightly together and season to taste with salt and freshly ground black pepper. Arrange the lettuce leaves on a platter. Pile the fish mixture on top and arrange the tomato slices and pepper rings around it. Serve garnished with the olives.

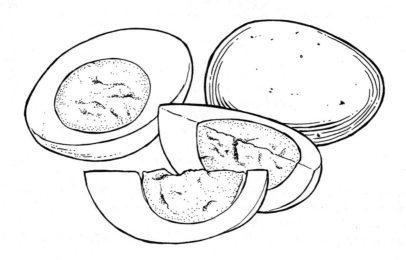

Sailor's Pie

Serves 4

1 tbs corn or sunflower oil
1 onion, peeled and sliced
2 sticks celery, sliced
50g (2 oz) button mushrooms, sliced
3 tomatoes, sliced
salt and freshly ground black pepper
350g (12 oz) white fish, cooked and flaked
2-3 drops Tabasco sauce
225g (8 oz) potatoes, peeled and thinly sliced

Heat the oil in a pan and sauté the onion and celery for 2-3 minutes. Add the mushrooms and tomatoes and cook for 3-4 minutes. Put half the mixture in an ovenproof casserole.

Season the fish to taste with salt and freshly ground black pepper and put it into the casserole, mixing it in together with the Tabasco sauce. Top with the remaining vegetables.

Arrange the sliced potatoes, in overlapping circles on top of the casserole and lay a piece of dampened greaseproof paper over them. Cover with foil and bake at 350°F/180°C (Gas Mark 4) for approximately 1 hour. Then remove the foil and paper and cook under a grill for 2-3 minutes to brown the potatoes. Serve immediately.

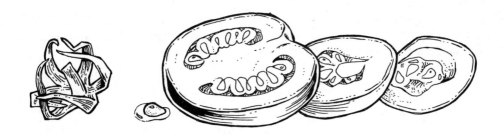

Fish

Haddock Crumble

Serves 4

450g (1 lb) haddock
275ml (½ pt) skimmed milk
1 tbs corn or sunflower oil
1 onion, peeled and chopped
2 tsp curry powder
25g (1 oz) flour
1 tbs sultanas
1 tbs mango chutney
50g (2 oz) frozen sweetcorn, cooked
salt and freshly ground black pepper

Crumble topping
25g (1 oz) porridge oats
25g (1 oz) wholemeal flour
25g (1 oz) low-fat spread
1 tbs fresh parsley, chopped
salt and freshly ground black pepper

Put the fish and milk in a pan and poach for 10-15 minutes, then drain off the liquid and reserve it. Flake the fish, removing any bones or skin, and put it in a lightly greased ovenproof dish.

Heat the oil in a pan and sauté the onion. Stir in the curry powder and flour and cook, stirring, for 1 minute. Stir in the milk and bring to the boil, stirring until it is thick and smooth. Add the sultanas, chutney and sweetcorn. Season to taste with salt and freshly ground black pepper, then pour the sauce over the fish.

To make the topping, put the oats and flour in a bowl. Rub in the low-fat spread, then stir in the parsley and seasoning. Spoon it evenly over the fish and cook in the oven at 350°F/180°C (Gas Mark 4) for 40 minutes. Serve immediately.

Steamed Trout with Yogurt Sauce

CHO 10g
Kcals 750

Serves 4

4 trout (each about 175g/6 oz), gutted and cleaned
4 tbs lemon juice
1 tbs fresh parsley, chopped
freshly ground black pepper

Yogurt sauce
1×150-g (5-fl oz) carton low-fat natural yogurt
1 tbs horseradish sauce
2 tbs lemon juice
1-2 tsp fresh chives, chopped
pinch cayenne pepper

Put the trout on a large sheet of foil and season with the lemon juice, parsley and pepper. Fold the foil loosely round the fish to form a parcel and steam for 10 to 15 minutes, or until fish flakes easily when tested with a fork.

Meanwhile, to make the sauce, put all the ingredients in a heatproof bowl. Put it over a pan of simmering water and stir until it is hot and creamy. Remove the trout from the foil and serve immediately with the yogurt sauce poured over them.

Stuffed Plaice

Serves 4

8 medium plaice fillets, skinned
3 tbs unsweetened apple juice
1 tbs soy sauce

Stuffing
50g (2 oz) wholemeal breadcrumbs
1-2 cloves garlic, crushed
1 small onion, peeled and finely chopped
25g (1 oz) ground almonds
½ tsp ground ginger
2 tbs unsweetened apple juice
1 tbs soy sauce
freshly ground black pepper

Lay the fillets flesh-side down on a clean surface. To make the stuffing, put all the ingredients in a bowl and mix them together well. Divide the stuffing between the fillets and roll up, securing them with cocktail sticks. Put the rolls in a shallow, lightly greased ovenproof dish.

Mix together the apple juice and soy sauce and pour this over the rolled fish. Cover with foil and cook at 350°F/180°C (Gas Mark 4) for 30 minutes. Serve immediately.

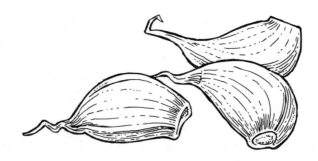

Haddock and
Vegetable Casserole

CHO 40g
Kcals 720

Serves 4

1 tbs corn or sunflower oil
1 onion, peeled and sliced
1 green pepper, deseeded and chopped
3 tomatoes, chopped
1 tsp oregano
225g (8 oz) potatoes, peeled and cubed
1 tbs tomato purée
salt and freshly ground black pepper
450g (1 lb) haddock fillet, skinned and cut into large pieces
3 tbs lemon juice
2 courgettes, sliced

Heat the oil in a pan and sauté the onion and pepper for 2-3 minutes. Add the tomatoes, oregano, potatoes, tomato purée and season to taste with salt and freshly ground black pepper. Bring to the boil, cover and simmer for 20 minutes, until the potatoes are just tender.

Meanwhile, put the fish and lemon juice in a bowl and season. Mix them together well, then add them to the pan, along with the courgettes, cover and simmer for 10 minutes until the fish is tender. Serve immediately.

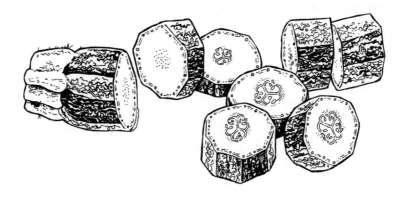

Fish

Baked Fish with Pepper Sauce

CHO neg
Kcals 910

Serves 4

4 cod or haddock fillets (each about 175g/6 oz)
25g (1 oz) low-fat spread, melted
4 tbs lemon juice
salt and freshly ground black pepper

Pepper sauce
1 tbs corn or sunflower oil
2 red peppers, deseeded and chopped
1 small onion, peeled and chopped
2 tbs single cream
lemon twists to garnish

Put the fish in a lightly greased baking dish and brush with the melted low-fat spread. Drizzle with the lemon juice and season to taste with salt and freshly ground black pepper. Cover with foil and cook at 350°F/180°C (Gas Mark 4) for 20-25 minutes, until tender.

Meanwhile, make the sauce. Heat the oil, add the pepper and onion and cook for 5 minutes. Add 3 tbs of water, bring to the boil, cover and cook gently for 10-15 minutes. Transfer the sauce to a blender and process until smooth. Return it to the pan, stir in the cream and season to taste. Reheat it gently, then serve the fish on warmed serving plates and with the sauce, garnished with the lemon twists.

Haddock and Spinach Bake

CHO 40g
Kcals 960

Serves 4

450g (1 lb) frozen spinach, cooked
450g (1 lb) haddock fillet, skinned and cut into pieces
1 tbs corn or sunflower oil
1 onion, chopped
2 celery sticks, chopped
1 pepper, deseeded and chopped
350g (12 oz) tomatoes, chopped
1 tbs tomato purée
1 glass dry white wine
5 tbs vegetable stock
salt and freshly ground black pepper
225g (8 oz) potatoes, cooked and thinly sliced

Preheat the oven to 375°F/190°C (Gas Mark 5), then lay the spinach leaves over the bottom of a lightly greased ovenproof dish and put the fish on top of it.

Heat the oil in a pan and sauté the onion and celery until they have softened. Add the pepper and tomatoes and stir well. Add the tomato purée, wine and stock and bring to the boil. Simmer for 5 minutes, then season to taste with salt and freshly ground black pepper.

Pour the vegetable mixture over the fish and arrange the potatoes over the top. Cook the dish in the preheated oven for 30 minutes until the potatoes are golden brown.

Fish

Rice with Prawns

Serves 6

2 tbs corn or sunflower oil
1 onion, peeled and chopped
1 clove garlic, crushed
1 tsp ground coriander
1 tsp ground cumin
1 tsp curry powder
175g (6 oz) frozen prawns, thawed
1 tbs soy sauce
100g (4 oz) frozen peas, cooked
salt and freshly ground black pepper
175g (6 oz) brown rice, cooked
3 spring onions, chopped

Heat the oil, add the onion and garlic and fry until they have softened. Add the coriander, cumin and curry powder and stir until they are well combined. Stir in the prawns until they are coated in the spices. Add the soy sauce, peas, 4 tbs of water and season to taste with salt and freshly ground black pepper. Cook the mixture for 2 minutes, then add the rice and mix everything together thoroughly. Cover and cook gently until it has heated through. Turn the mixture onto a warmed serving dish, sprinkle the spring onions over it and serve immediately.

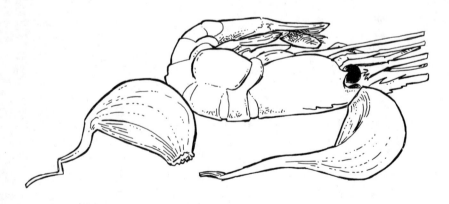

Mackerel with
Mustard and Oats

CHO 10g
Kcals 1650

Serves 4

4 mackerel fillets (each about 175g/6 oz)
1 tbs lemon juice
salt and freshly ground black pepper
2 tsp made mustard
25g (1 oz) porridge oats

Put the mackerel on a grill rack lined with foil. Drizzle the lemon juice over the fish and season with salt and freshly ground black pepper.

Stir the mustard and oats together and spread the mixture over the mackerel. Cook the fish under a medium-hot grill for 10-15 minutes, then serve immediately.

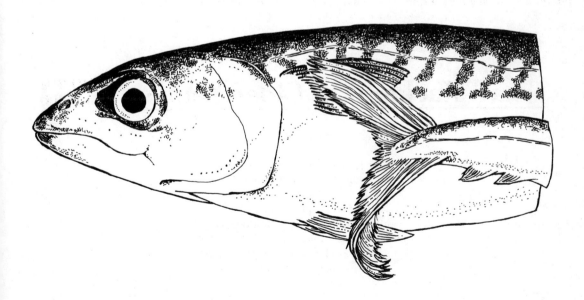

Fish Creole

Serves 4

1 onion, peeled and chopped
1 green pepper, deseeded and chopped
1×400-g (14-oz) tin chopped tomatoes
pinch basil
pinch oregano
salt and freshly ground black pepper
225g (8 oz) white fish, cut into cubes
225g (8 oz) frozen prawns, defrosted
1 tsp cornflour
2 tbs dry white wine
fresh parsley, chopped, to garnish

Put the onion, pepper, tomatoes and herbs and seasoning in a pan and bring to the boil. Cover and simmer for 10 minutes. Add the fish and prawns and simmer for a further 10-15 minutes.

Blend the cornflour with the wine, then stir this mixture into the sauce and stir for 1-2 minutes while it thickens. Serve immediately, garnished with the chopped parsley.

Mackerel in Cider Sauce

Serves 4

1 tbs corn or sunflower oil
1 onion, peeled and chopped
1 tbs flour
275ml (½ pt) dry cider
salt and freshly ground black pepper
4 mackerel (each about 175g/6 oz), filleted
1 eating apple, peeled, cored and finely sliced
fresh parsley, chopped

Heat the oil and sauté the onion until it is soft. Add the flour and cook for 2 minutes, stirring constantly. Stir in the cider and season to taste with salt and freshly ground black pepper. Add the mackerel fillets, cover the pan and simmer gently for 15 minutes, or until the mackerel is tender.

Then transfer the mackerel to a warmed serving dish and keep warm. Add the apples to the sauce and simmer until the sauce has reduced and is the consistency of double cream. Pour it over the fish and sprinkle the parsley over it. Serve immediately.

Cod Bake

CHO 30g
Kcals 990

Serves 4

1×275-g/10-oz packet frozen chopped spinach, cooked according to instructions on packet
pinch freshly grated nutmeg
salt and freshly ground black pepper
4 cod steaks
25g (1 oz) low-fat spread

Sauce
25g (1 oz) low-fat spread
25g (1 oz) flour
275ml (½ pt) skimmed milk
50g (2 oz) reduced-fat cheddar cheese, grated
salt and freshly ground black pepper

Season the spinach with the nutmeg, salt and pepper and lay it in the bottom of a shallow ovenproof dish. Then poach the cod steaks gently in the low-fat spread and put them on top of the spinach in the dish.

To prepare the sauce, melt the low-fat spread in a pan, stir in the flour and cook for 1-2 minutes, stirring constantly. Remove the pan from the heat and add the milk gradually. Return the pan to the heat and bring the sauce to the boil, stirring constantly. Reduce the heat, stir in half the cheese and season to taste with salt and freshly ground black pepper.

Cover the fish with the cheese sauce and sprinkle the remaining cheese over the top. Bake for 20-30 minutes at 375°F/190°C (Gas Mark 5), or until the fish is cooked. Serve immediately.

Fish Steaks and Peppercorn Sauce

CHO 20g
Kcals 1500

Serves 6

6 white fish steaks or cutlets
25g (1 oz) flour
salt and freshly ground black pepper

Peppercorn sauce
2 tbs corn or sunflower oil
1 wine glass of red wine
150ml (¼ pt) fish stock
1×150-ml (5-fl oz) carton single cream
2 tomatoes, chopped
2 tsp peppercorns, crushed

Coat the fish with the flour, to which salt and pepper have been added. Heat the oil in a frying pan and cook the fish for about 5 minutes on each side until it is just tender. Remove the fish to a heated serving dish and keep it warm.

Add the wine to the juices in the pan, scraping the pan to ensure that all the sediment is incorporated into the sauce. Boil until the wine has reduced to 3 tbs. Add the stock, stir well and boil until it has reduced to half the original quantity. Add the cream and stir over a low heat (do not boil or the cream will curdle) until the sauce is smooth. Add the tomatoes and peppercorns and adjust the seasoning if necessary. Heat until the sauce is just about to boil, then pour it over the fish and serve immediately.

Fish Pie

Serves 2

350g (12 oz) cod fillets, skinned and boned
15g (½ oz) low-fat spread
salt and freshly ground black pepper

Topping
2 medium-sized potatoes (each about 225g/8 oz), peeled and cooked
a little low-fat spread
a little skimmed milk
salt and freshly ground black pepper

Sauce
15g (½ oz) low-fat spread
15g (½ oz) flour
150ml (¼ pt) skimmed milk
1 tsp anchovy essence (optional)
1 tbs parsley, finely chopped

Put the fish in an ovenproof dish and spread the low-fat spread over it. Season to taste with salt and freshly ground black pepper. Cover and bake at 325°F/170°C (Gas Mark 3) for 20-30 minutes or until the fish flakes easily. Strain off the fish liquor and reserve it for the sauce.

Meanwhile, cream the potatoes with the low-fat spread, milk and season.

To make the sauce, melt the low-fat spread in a pan and blend in the flour. Add enough milk to the reserved fish liquor to make it up to 275ml (½ pt), then blend it gradually with the spread and flour to make a smooth sauce. Bring it to the boil and simmer for 3 minutes, stirring continuously.

Blend the anchovy essence and flaked fish into the sauce and season to taste. Turn the mixture into an ovenproof dish, spread the prepared mashed potato over the fish and bake at 400°F/200°C (Gas Mark 6) for 20 minutes or until the top is golden brown.

Fish

Summer Fish

Serves 4

salt and freshly ground black pepper
4 white fish fillets
4 rashers lean streaky bacon
25g (1 oz) low-fat spread
3 courgettes, sliced
pinch tarragon
3 tbs dry vermouth
150ml (5 fl oz) single cream

Season the fish with salt and freshly ground black pepper and wrap a bacon rasher around each fillet, then put them in a lightly greased baking dish. Dot them with the low-fat spread. Arrange the courgettes around the fish and sprinkle the tarragon over them. Mix the vermouth and cream together and pour it over the fish. Cover the dish and bake at 350°F/180°C (Gas Mark 4) for 20 minutes or until the fish is tender.

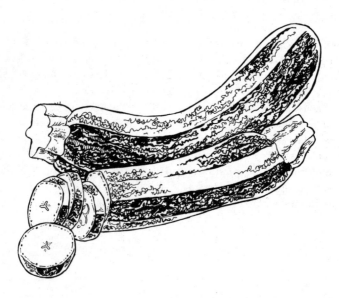

Steamed Fish
and Vegetables

CHO neg
Kcals 1550

Serves 6

25g (1 oz) low-fat spread
1 tbs olive or sunflower oil
1 onion, sliced
4 carrots, cut into julienne
3 sticks celery, cut into thin strips
1 bulb fennel, cut into thin strips
1 wineglass dry white wine
150ml (¼ pt) fish stock
pinch mixed herbs
salt and freshly ground black pepper
approximately 900g (2 lb) halibut on the bone
150ml (5 fl oz) single cream

Heat the low-fat spread and oil in a shallow pan large enough to accommodate the fish and that has a tight-fitting lid. Add the onion, carrots, celery and fennel and cook for 2-3 minutes. Add the wine and bring it to the boil for 3 minutes to reduce it. Then add the stock, herbs and seasonings. Put the fish on top of the vegetables, cover and steam it over a low heat for about 20 minutes until the fish is cooked. Remove the fish, put the vegetables onto a warmed serving dish and place the fish on top. Add the cream to the juices and heat it through without boiling it (otherwise it will curdle). Pour the sauce over the fish and serve immediately.

Fish

Fish-based Pizza

Serves 4

4 white fish steaks
2 tomatoes, sliced
4 lean rashers streaky bacon, cut into long strips
pinch oregano
salt and freshly ground black pepper
4 stuffed olives, sliced
1 tbs olive oil
50g (2 oz) reduced-fat cheddar cheese, sliced

Put the fish in a lightly greased baking dish and cover with the slices of tomato, then make a lattice pattern with the bacon. Sprinkle the oregano over the top and season with salt and freshly ground black pepper. Put the olive slices in the lattice and brush the whole design with oil. Lay the slices of cheese over the top. Bake at 375°F/190°C (Gas Mark 5) for about 20 minutes until the fish is cooked.

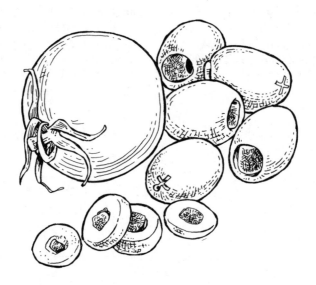

Fish Chowder

Serves 4-6

2 tbs olive oil
1 onion, chopped
1 clove garlic, crushed
1×400-g (14-oz) tin chopped tomatoes
1 carrot, chopped
225g (8 oz) potato, peeled and diced
450g (1 lb) white fish, cut into bite-size pieces
550ml (1 pt) water
freshly ground black pepper
275ml (½ pt) skimmed milk
fresh parsley, chopped, to garnish

Heat the oil in a pan and add all the vegetables, except the potato, and cook for 5 minutes. Add the potato, fish, water and pepper and bring to the boil, skimming off any froth. Cover and simmer gently for 20-30 minutes or until the vegetables are tender. Add the milk and heat gently. Adjust the seasoning to taste and serve garnished with the parsley.

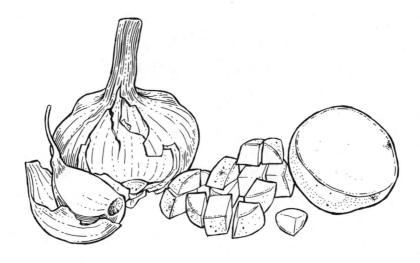

Salmon Parcels

Serves 4

4 salmon steaks
25g (1 oz) low-fat spread
4 bay leaves
4 sprigs parsley
1 onion, quartered
4 slices lemon
salt and freshly ground black pepper

Put each salmon steak on a square of foil and dot each one with the low-fat spread. Top with a bay leaf, a sprig of parsley, quarter of onion, slice of lemon and seasonings. Wrap the steaks in the foil and put the parcels in an ovenproof dish. Barely cover the bottom of the dish with water and bake at 350°F/180°C (Gas Mark 4) for 15-20 minutes or until the salmon is tender. Serve immediately.

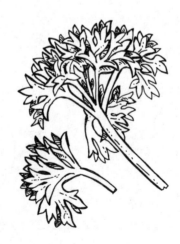

Fish Cakes

Make 4

225g (8 oz) smoked haddock, cooked and flaked
225g (8 oz) potatoes, boiled and mashed
1 tbs fresh parsley, chopped
1 tsp lemon juice
salt and freshly ground black pepper
a little olive or sunflower oil for frying

Coating
1 × size 3 egg, beaten
50g (2 oz) wholemeal breadcrumbs

In a bowl, mix the fish, potatoes, parsley, lemon juice and salt and pepper, binding them together with 1 tbs milk if needed. Shape them into 4 cakes and dip them in the beaten egg, then coat them in the breadcrumbs.

Heat the oil (about 3 tbs should be enough) and fry the fish cakes for 5-7 minutes on each side or until they are golden brown then serve.

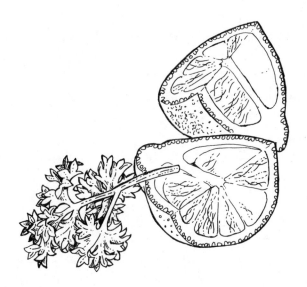

Fish

Vegetarian Dishes

Vegetarian meals generally contain more protein and fibre than meat or fish-based meals, so are more colourful and have wonderful texture. Also, as meat is the most expensive ingredient, they are more economical. Pasta, rice, beans and other pulses are ideal for fast meals as they are quick to prepare and very versatile when combined with different sauces or fillings.

Whether you are vegetarian or not, the recipes in this section are tasty and healthy ways to increase your intake of fibre and reduce the amount of fat you eat, so eating vegetarian regularly is definitely a good idea.

Pasta and Pesto Sauce

Serves 4

75g (3 oz) fresh or 5 tbs dried basil
50g (2 oz) pine nuts
2-3 cloves garlic, crushed
¼ tsp salt
freshly ground black pepper
150ml (¼ pt) olive or rapeseed oil
2 tbs Parmesan cheese, finely grated
175g-225g (6-8 oz) wholewheat pasta, cooked

Put the basil, pine nuts, garlic and salt in a blender or food processor and blend for 1-2 minutes. Slowly add the oil, a little at a time, then stir in the cheese by hand. Toss it well with the freshly cooked *al dente* pasta.

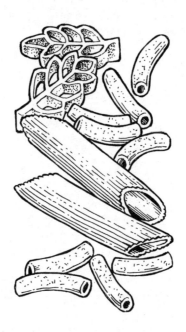

Vegetable Lasagne

Serves 4-6

Filling
1 tbs olive or sunflower oil
1 onion, sliced
1 clove garlic, crushed
1 green pepper, deseeded and chopped
2 medium carrots, peeled and thinly sliced
100g (4 oz) button mushrooms, sliced
1×400-g (14-oz) tin tomatoes
1 tsp mixed herbs
salt and freshly ground black pepper
225g (8 oz) frozen spinach, defrosted and drained
6 slices pre-cooked wholewheat lasagne

White sauce
15g (½ oz) polyunsaturated margarine
15g (½ oz) wholemeal flour
150ml (¼ pt) skimmed milk
25g (1 oz) reduced-fat or vegetarian cheddar cheese

Topping
25g (1 oz) reduced-fat cheddar cheese
25g (1 oz) unsalted cashew nuts

Heat the oil in a pan and lightly sauté the onion and garlic in the oil. Add the pepper, carrot and mushrooms and cook for about 5 minutes. Stir in the tomatoes, herbs and season to taste with salt and freshly ground black pepper. Allow to simmer for 5-10 minutes, stirring occasionally.

Meanwhile, make the white sauce. Melt the margarine, stir in the flour and cook for 1 minute. Gradually stir in the milk and bring to the boil, stirring continuously until the sauce has thickened. Stir in the cheese and season to taste.

Layer the bolognese mixture, with the spinach and lasagne sheets in alternate layers in an oblong dish, ending with a layer of lasagne. Cover the top with the cheese sauce and sprinkle with the cashew nuts and the remaining cheese. Bake at 350°F/180°C (Gas Mark 4) for 30-35 minutes.

Vegetarian Dishes

Red Lentil Lasagne

Serves 6

225g (8 oz) red lentils
1 tbs olive or sunflower oil
1 large onion, chopped
2 cloves garlic, crushed
1 green pepper, deseeded and chopped
100g (4 oz) mushrooms, sliced
1 tsp dried basil
1 tsp dried oregano
1 × 400-g (14-oz) tin chopped tomatoes
1 tsp yeast extract
275ml (½ pt) water
1 bay leaf
salt and freshly ground black pepper
8 sheets pre-cooked spinach lasagne (lasagne verde)

White sauce
25g (1 oz) low-fat spread
25g (1 oz) wholemeal flour
275ml (½ pt) skimmed milk
1 tsp mustard powder
salt and freshly ground black pepper
75g (3 oz) reduced-fat vegetarian cheese, grated

Bring the lentils to the boil in plenty of unsalted water. Boil them fast for 10 minutes, then drain them.

Heat the oil in a pan and gently fry the onion and garlic over a moderate heat for 5 minutes. Add the pepper and mushrooms and cook for 5 minutes, stirring from time to time.

Add the basil, oregano and drained lentils and cook gently for 2-3 minutes. Stir in the tomatoes and their juice, the yeast extract, water and bay leaf. Bring to the boil, cover and simmer for 15-20 minutes until the lentils are soft. Season with salt and freshly ground black pepper, then remove the bay leaf.

Next, make the white sauce. Melt the low-fat spread in a small pan and stir in the flour. Cook it over a gentle heat for 2-3 minutes, stirring. Remove the pan from the heat and gradually stir in the milk. Bring to the boil, stirring all the time, until the sauce thickens. Cook gently for 1-2 minutes. Remove the pan from the heat and beat in the mustard powder and season and a third of the cheese.

In a rectangular dish, layer the lentil sauce and lasagne sheets, finishing with a layer of lasagne.

Pour the cheese sauce over the top and sprinkle the remaining cheese over it.

Bake the lasagne in the oven at 350°F/180°C (Gas Mark 4) for 30-35 minutes until the cheese has melted, is bubbling and golden brown.

Leeks and Pasta

CHO neg
Kcals 350

Serves 4

1 tbs corn or sunflower oil
2 leeks, thinly sliced
100g (4 oz) button mushrooms
100g (4 oz) low-fat garlic and herb soft cheese
90ml (3 fl oz) skimmed milk

Bring a large pan of slightly salted water to the boil and cook the pasta until it is *al dente*.

Meanwhile, heat the oil in a pan and lightly fry the leeks and mushrooms until they have softened a little. Mix the cheese with the milk, then add it to the pan and heat gently to make a smooth, creamy sauce. Mix the sauce thoroughly with the pasta and serve straight away.

Note Remember to take into account the CHO values of any pasta — 45g cooked weight of wholemeal spaghetti = 10g CHO.

Vegetarian Paella

CHO 80g
Kcals 810

Serves 4

1 tbs olive or sunflower oil
2 onions, peeled and chopped
2 cloves of garlic, crushed
100g (4 oz) brown rice
275ml (½ pt) vegetable stock
pinch basil
2 courgettes, washed and sliced
1 red pepper, deseeded and sliced
1×227-g (8 oz) tin tomatoes
freshly ground black pepper
50g (2 oz) reduced-fat cheddar cheese, grated
15g (½ oz) flaked almonds

Heat the oil in a pan and add the onions and garlic. Add the rice and cook for a further few minutes coating the grains well with the oil. Add the stock and basil, bring to the boil, reduce the heat, cover and simmer for 25-30 minutes. Add the courgettes, pepper and tomatoes. Season with black pepper and cook for about 10 minutes until the rice is cooked and the vegetables are tender. Spoon the mixture into an ovenproof dish. Sprinkle the cheese and almonds over the top and grill until lightly browned. Serve immediately.

Rice and Millet Salad

Serves 6-8

100g (4 oz) long-grained brown rice
100g (4 oz) millet
1 onion, finely chopped
6 cardamom pods, slightly crushed
20 coriander seeds, crushed
pinch of cinnamon
425ml (¾ pt) vegetable stock
2 sprigs fresh thyme
salt and freshly ground black pepper
4 stalks celery, trimmed and cut into small chunks
1 red pepper, deseeded and diced
25g (1 oz) hazelnuts or walnuts, lightly toasted
1 tbs fresh coriander, roughly chopped

Dressing
1 tsp light soy sauce
2 tbs lemon juice

Wash the rice and millet and leave them to drain.

Meanwhile, sweat the onion and spices over gentle heat in a non-stick pan for 2-3 minutes. Add the rice and millet, stirring with a wooden spoon, then add the stock and thyme. Stir again to ensure that no grains have stuck to the bottom of the pan and season with salt and freshly ground black pepper. Bring to the boil, cover and simmer for about 20-25 minutes. The grains should now be tender and all the liquid should have been absorbed.

Tip the rice and millet into a warmed serving bowl and use a fork to separate the grains, removing the thyme and cardamom pods as you go. Leave it to cool before adding the celery, pepper, nuts and coriander. Mix the dressing and pour it over the salad. Mix everything together well and serve.

Vegetarian Dishes

Savoury Rice

Serves 6

2 tbs corn or sunflower oil
1 onion, chopped
1 clove garlic, crushed
½ red pepper, chopped
225g (8 oz) brown rice, cooked
1×size 3 egg, beaten
2 tsp soy sauce
salt and freshly ground black pepper

Heat the oil in a frying pan and sauté the onion, garlic and pepper for 5 minutes. Add the rice and stir for 2-3 minutes. Stir in the beaten egg and soy sauce, stirring until the egg is distributed throughout the rice and lightly cooked. Season to taste with salt and freshly ground black pepper before serving.

Three-bean Cassoulet

Serves 4

1 onion, peeled and sliced
1 clove garlic, crushed
1×400-g (14-oz) tin flageolet beans, drained
1×225-g (8-oz) tin red kidney beans, drained and refreshed under
cold running water
100g (4 oz) cut green beans, cooked
1×225-g (8-oz) tin tomatoes
pinch mixed herbs
salt and freshly ground black pepper
150ml (¼ pt) vegetable stock
25g (1 oz) sunflower seeds, toasted

Put all the ingredients, except the sunflower seeds, into a flameproof casserole and bring to the boil. Simmer for about 20 minutes, stirring occasionally. Sprinkle the sunflower seeds over the top just before you serve.

Bean and Vegetable Stew

CHO 100g
Kcals 1020

Serves 4-6

1 tbs corn or sunflower oil
2 cloves garlic, crushed
450g (1 lb) leeks, sliced
1 large carrot, sliced
225g (8 oz) mushrooms, sliced
1 tbs paprika
1 tbs light soy sauce
275ml (½ pt) vegetable stock
1×225-g (8-oz) tin red kidney beans, drained and refreshed under cold running water
salt and freshly ground black pepper

Dumplings
100g (4 oz) self-raising 100 per cent wholemeal flour
50g (2 oz) vegetable suet
pinch salt
1 tbs parsley, chopped
a little water to bind

Heat the oil in a flameproof casserole. Add the garlic, leeks, carrot and mushrooms and sauté them until they are tender. Add the paprika, soy sauce and stock and bring to the boil. Add the kidney beans, salt and freshly ground black pepper and simmer for 20 minutes.

Meanwhile, make the dumplings. Mix all the ingredients together to make a firm dough. Shape it into 6-8 dumplings and arrange them on top of the stew. Cover the casserole and simmer gently for 20 minutes until the dumplings are light and fluffy, then serve straight away.

Vegetarian Dishes

Chick Pea Moussaka

CHO 160g
Kcals 1270

Serves 4

1 large aubergine
350g (12 oz) potatoes, peeled
1 onion, peeled and finely chopped
2 cloves garlic, crushed
1 tbs olive or sunflower oil
50g (2 oz) mushrooms, sliced
1×400-g (14-oz) tin chopped tomatoes
2 tsp dried oregano
1 tbs Worcestershire sauce
dash of Tabasco sauce
1×400-g (14-oz) tin chick peas, drained
sea salt and freshly ground black pepper

Topping
2×size 3 eggs, beaten
1 tsp cumin seeds, toasted (optional)
1×150-g (5-fl oz) carton low-fat natural yogurt
tomato slices and parsley, to garnish

Prick and trim the aubergines and bake them in a 350°F/180°C (Gas Mark 4) oven for 20-30 minutes, then slice (leaving the oven on). Boil the potatoes until they are tender, then slice them thickly. Gently fry the onion and garlic in the oil for 4-5 minutes. Add the mushrooms, tomatoes, oregano, Worcestershire and Tabasco sauces, chick peas and season with salt and freshly ground black pepper. Cook gently for 10 minutes, adjusting the seasoning if necessary.

Arrange layers of aubergine, potato and vegetable sauce in an ovenproof casserole dish, finishing with a layer of aubergine. Beat together the topping ingredients and spoon the mixture over the moussaka. Bake in the oven for 25-30 minutes.

Mixed Bean Hot Pot

Serves 3-4

1×225g (8 oz) tin cannellini beans, drained and rinsed
100g (4 oz) French beans
1×225-g (8-oz) tin tomatoes
1 tbs tomato purée
1 clove garlic, crushed
1 tsp mixed herbs
salt and freshly ground black pepper
225g (8 oz) potatoes, parboiled and thinly sliced
25g (1 oz) reduced-fat vegetarian cheddar cheese, grated

Mix all the ingredients together, except the potatoes and cheese, and pour it into an ovenproof dish. Arrange the sliced potatoes on top of the mixture and sprinkle the cheese over them. Cook at 325°F/170°C (Gas Mark 3) for 45 minutes-1 hour or until the potatoes are cooked.

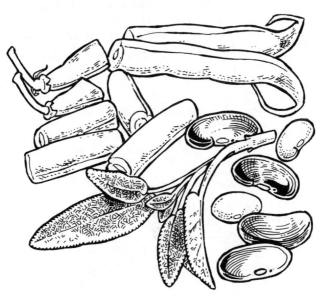

Braised Green Lentils

CHO 110g
Kcals 990

This mixture can be used to make a vegetarian Shepherd's Pie by piping creamed potato over the top.

Serves 4

225g (8 oz) green lentils
1 tbs olive or sunflower oil
1 onion, peeled and finely chopped
1 small potato, cut into small pieces
1 carrot, scrubbed and diced
1 leek, washed and finely sliced
2 tomatoes, seeded and diced
275ml (½ pt) vegetable stock
1 small garlic clove, crushed
salt and freshly ground black pepper
1 tsp white wine vinegar

Wash the lentils thoroughly and leave to drain. Heat the oil in a pan and sauté the remaining vegetables gently, stirring all the time, for about 3-4 minutes. Add the stock, garlic and drained lentils and bring to the boil. Simmer until the lentils are just tender (about 7-10 minutes). Season to taste with salt and freshly ground black pepper and add the vinegar.

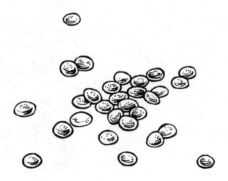

Lentil Moussaka

Serves 6

2 medium aubergines, sliced
2 tbs olive oil
2 medium onions, peeled and chopped
100g (4 oz) green lentils, cooked
1 tsp mixed herbs
1 tsp nutmeg, grated
1 tbs tomato purée
1×400-g (14-oz) tin tomatoes, drained and chopped, reserving the juice
2 medium potatoes, boiled with their skins on, then sliced

White sauce
25g (1 oz) low-fat spread
25g (1 oz) flour
275ml (½ pt) skimmed milk
1×size 3 egg
salt and freshly ground black pepper
½ tsp nutmeg, grated
1 tomato, sliced

Sprinkle the aubergine slices with salt and leave to stand for 30 minutes to remove the bitter juices. Pat dry with kitchen paper towels. Then heat the oil in a pan and fry the aubergines until they are golden brown. Set aside.

Fry the onions in the pan until they are soft, then add the lentils, herbs, nutmeg, tomato purée and tomato juice. Simmer for 5 minutes.

Assemble the moussaka by arranging a layer of aubergine slices in an ovenproof dish, followed by slices of potato, chopped tomatoes and the lentil texture. Repeat until all ingredients are used, ending with a layer of aubergine slices.

To make the sauce, melt the low-fat spread in a pan, stir in the flour, then gradually add the milk. Bring to the boil, stirring all the time, then reduce the heat and simmer for 2-3 minutes until the sauce is thickened, stirring continuously. Remove the pan from the heat, season to taste and allow to cool slightly before beating in the egg quickly until the sauce is glossy. Pour the sauce over the moussaka. Garnish with the sliced tomato. Bake at 375°F/190°C (Gas Mark 5) for 45 minutes and serve hot.

Mung Bean and
Vegetable Cottage Pie

CHO 190g
Kcals 1220

Serves 4-6

2 tsp sunflower oil
1 onion, finely chopped
2 carrots, finely chopped
3 sticks celery, diced
225g (8 oz) mung beans, cooked
2 tsp cayenne pepper
1 tsp fresh marjoram, chopped
1 tsp fresh sage, chopped
1 tbs tomato purée
1 tsp yeast extract
275ml (½ pt) vegetable stock
salt and freshly ground black pepper
450g (1 lb) potatoes, peeled and diced
4 tbs skimmed milk
15g (½ oz) sunflower seeds

Preheat the oven to 350°F/180°C (Gas Mark 4).

Heat the oil in a large pan and fry the onion, carrots and celery for 5 minutes. Add the cooked mung beans, cayenne pepper, herbs, tomato purée, yeast extract and stock. Cover and simmer gently for 10-15 minutes. Season to taste with salt and freshly ground black pepper.

Meanwhile, boil the potatoes until they are cooked. Drain and mash them with the milk. Put the bean mixture into a large casserole dish and top this with the mashed potato. Sprinkle the sunflower seeds over the top and bake in the preheated oven for 30-40 minutes, until the top is golden brown.

Courgette and Sweetcorn Gratin

CHO 110g
Kcals 1100

Serves 4-6

100g (4 oz) red lentils
2 tsp olive or sunflower oil
1 onion, peeled and finely chopped
1 clove garlic, crushed
1 tbs tomato purée
50g (2 oz) oatmeal
1 tbs lemon juice
1 tsp dried mixed herbs
salt and freshly ground black pepper

Filling
100g (4 oz) courgettes, finely diced
100g (4 oz) red pepper, deseeded and finely diced
1×size 3 egg, beaten
1 tbs wholemeal flour
100ml (4 fl oz) skimmed milk
100g (4 oz) tinned sweetcorn
salt and freshly ground black pepper
50g (2 oz) vegetarian cheese, grated

Boil the lentils in plenty of unsalted water. Boil them fast for 10 minutes then drain them well.

Heat the oil in a pan and gently fry the onion for 2-3 minutes. Add the garlic and fry it for 1 minute. Remove the pan from the heat and mix in the lentils, tomato purée, oatmeal, lemon juice and herbs. Season to taste with salt and freshly ground black pepper. The mixture should be thick enough to hold together, but if the lentils are still a little wet, return the pan to the heat to dry it out a little, stirring, or add a little more oatmeal. Press the mixture around the sides and bottom of a 20-cm/8-inch flan dish.

For the filling, lightly steam the courgettes and pepper for 4 minutes or until tender. Blend the egg with the flour, then add the milk. Stir in the cooked courgettes and sweetcorn and season well. Spoon the filling into the flan dish, cover the top with the cheese. Bake at 375°F/190°C (Gas Mark 5) for 30-35 minutes, or until the filling has set and serve hot.

Vegetarian Dishes

Stuffed Mushrooms

CHO 30g
Kcals 400

Serves 4

4 large field mushrooms
50g (2 oz) wholemeal breadcrumbs
50g (2 oz) reduced-fat cheddar cheese, grated
25g (1 oz) walnuts, finely chopped
pinch mixed herbs
freshly ground black pepper
1 tbs tomato ketchup

Remove the mushroom stalks and chop them finely. Mix them together with the remaining ingredients. Spoon equal amounts into each of the mushroom caps and put them on a baking sheet. Bake them at 375°F/190°C (Gas Mark 5) for 10 minutes. Serve as soon as they are done.

Stir-fried Vegetables

CHO neg
Kcals 400

Serves 4

1 tbs olive or sunflower oil
4 carrots, cut into strips
half a cauliflower, broken into florets
175g (6 oz) baby sweetcorn
100g (4 oz) runner beans, cut into pieces
100g (4 oz) button mushrooms, sliced
225g (8 oz) beansprouts
2 tsp soy sauce

Heat the oil in a wok or large frying pan. Add the carrots, cauliflower, sweetcorn and beans and stir for 1-2 minutes. Add the remaining vegetables and cook 1-2 more minutes. Toss the vegetables in the soy sauce and serve immediately.

Vegetable Casserole

CHO 10g
Kcals 190

Serves 4

1 small swede (about 225g/8 oz), peeled and finely diced
2 carrots, peeled and sliced
1 large onion, peeled and sliced
4 sticks celery, chopped
1×400-g (14-oz) tin tomatoes
salt and freshly ground black pepper
pinch ground nutmeg
about 150ml (¼ pt) vegetable stock

Mix the prepared vegetables together in a 1.75l (3-pt) casserole dish. Season to taste with salt and freshly ground black pepper. Pour the tomatoes and some of the stock over the vegetables and cook at 350°F/180°C (Gas Mark 4) for 1-1¼ hours, or until the vegetables are tender. Add some extra stock if the mixture begins to get a little dry.

Peppers à la Provence

CHO neg
Kcals 260

Serves 4

1 tbs olive or sunflower oil
2 medium onions, peeled and sliced
1 clove garlic, crushed
4 peppers (assorted colours), deseeded and sliced
1×400-g (14-oz) tin tomatoes
1 tsp *herbs de Provence*
salt and freshly ground black pepper

Heat the oil in a large pan, add the onions and garlic and fry them until they are soft. Add the peppers and cook for 5-10 minutes. Stir in the tomatoes, herbs and season to taste with salt and freshly ground black pepper. Bring to the boil, then simmer for 15-20 minutes. Serve either hot or cold.

Sautéed Okra

Serves 4

1 tbs olive or sunflower oil
1 onion, peeled and chopped
½ tsp chilli powder
1 tsp ground coriander
1 tsp garam masala
225g (8 oz) okra
1-2 tbs lemon juice
pinch of salt

Heat the oil in a pan and fry the onion, chilli powder, coriander and garam masala. Add the okra and lemon juice and a pinch of salt and cook for approximately 5 minutes. Serve immediately.

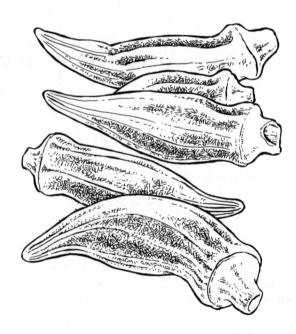

Cheesy Leek and Potato Casserole

CHO 110g
Kcals 930

Serves 4-6

450g (1 lb) leeks, sliced
1 onion, peeled and finely sliced
450g (1 lb) potatoes, thickly sliced
25g (1 oz) low-fat spread
25g (1 oz) wholemeal flour
275ml (½ pt) skimmed milk
½ tsp mustard
sea salt
½ tsp paprika
½ tsp ground cumin
50g (2 oz) vegetarian cheese, grated
½ tsp cumin seeds (optional)

Preheat the oven to 350°F/180°C (Gas Mark 4).

Steam the leeks over a large pan of simmering water for 8 minutes.

Meanwhile, cover the potato slices with water, bring to the boil and simmer gently for 8 minutes. Drain well.

While the potatoes are cooking, melt the low-fat spread in a pan, add the flour and cook gently, stirring, for 2-3 minutes. Remove the pan from the heat and gradually stir in the milk. Return the pan to the heat, bring the sauce to the boil, stirring constantly, and cook gently for 2-3 minutes. Stir in the mustard, seasoning and spices.

Layer the leek, onion and potato slices in a casserole or ovenproof dish. Pour the sauce over them and top with the grated cheese. Sprinkle the cumin seeds over, if using. Bake in the preheated oven for 30 minutes, or until the top is golden brown and the vegetables are cooked.

Vegetarian Dishes

Mixed Vegetable Curry

CHO 40g
Kcals 470

Serves 4-6

2 tsp olive or sunflower oil
1 tsp cumin seeds
1 tsp coriander seeds
1 large onion, peeled and finely chopped
3 cloves garlic, crushed
1 tsp garam masala
½ tsp chilli powder
1 medium potato, finely diced
100g (4 oz) cauliflower, cut into florets
2 courgettes, sliced
1 leek, sliced
1 green pepper, deseeded and cut into strips
25g (1 oz) wholemeal flour
1×400-g (14-oz) tin chopped tomatoes
150ml (¼ pt) vegetable stock
2 tbs low-fat natural yogurt
salt and freshly ground black pepper

Heat the oil in a large pan and gently cook the cumin and coriander seeds for 3-4 minutes until the seeds are turning brown. Then add the onion, garlic, garam masala and chilli powder and cook gently for 2 minutes. Add the potato, cauliflower, courgette, leek and green pepper and continue cooking for 3 minutes, stirring well to ensure that the vegetables are well coated in spices. Sprinkle the flour over them and cook for 1 minute. Add the tomatoes and their juice together with the stock. Bring to the boil, cover and simmer gently for 40-45 minutes, stirring occasionally, adding a little extra stock if the sauce thickens a little too much. When the vegetables are tender, add the yogurt. Adjust the seasoning to taste and serve hot.

COOK'S TIP
The flavours of the curry will have more time to develop if the dish is made a day in advance. 1-2 tablespoons of curry powder may be used in place of the various spices if you do not have them.

Stuffed Aubergines

Serves 6

3 medium aubergines
1 tbs olive or sunflower oil
2 large onions, peeled and chopped
2 cloves garlic, crushed
100g (4 oz) mushrooms, chopped
4 large tomatoes, skinned and chopped
1 tsp tomato purée
50g (2 oz) wholemeal breadcrumbs
2 tbs bran
25g (1 oz) blanched almonds, chopped
1 tbs fresh parsley, chopped
1 tsp lemon juice
salt and freshly ground black pepper
50g (2 oz) vegetarian cheese, grated

Prick the aubergines with a fork to prevent the skins from bursting, put them on a baking tray and bake them for 30 minutes at 350°F/180°C (Gas Mark 4), turning them once. Cut them in half lengthways and scoop out the flesh, leaving some to form thick skins for the shells. Chop the flesh.

Heat the oil in a pan and fry the onions and garlic over a moderate heat for 2 minutes, stirring occasionally. Add the mushrooms, tomatoes and tomato purée to the pan. Simmer for 5 minutes stirring occasionally, then add the chopped aubergine flesh, two-thirds of the breadcrumbs, half the bran, the almonds, parsley and lemon juice and season to taste with salt and freshly ground black pepper. Stir them all together well and simmer for 2-3 minutes.

Put the aubergine shells in an ovenproof dish and spoon the filling into the shells. Mix together the remaining breadcrumbs, bran and the cheese and sprinkle this over the tops of the aubergine shells, pressing down firmly on the filling. Bake for 20-25 minutes, until the cheese is bubbling and golden brown. Serve hot.

Serves 3

1 tbs olive oil or sunflower oil
1 clove garlic, crushed
1 small piece root ginger, peeled and crushed
½ tsp coriander seed, crushed
1 medium onion, peeled and chopped
100g (4 oz) baby sweetcorn, trimmed
3 small courgettes, cut into wedges
1 small red pepper, deseeded and sliced
1 small green pepper, deseeded and sliced
salt and freshly ground black pepper
1 tbs light soy sauce
1 tsp fresh coriander leaves to garnish

Heat the oil in a wok or large frying pan with a close-fitting lid. Add the garlic, ginger and coriander seed and cook for a minute. Add the onion, sweetcorn and courgettes. Cover and cook for a few minutes. Add the peppers, cover and cook for 5 minutes, stirring occasionally. Season with salt and freshly ground black pepper. Remove the pan from the heat and add the soy sauce. Serve warm, garnished with the fresh coriander leaves.

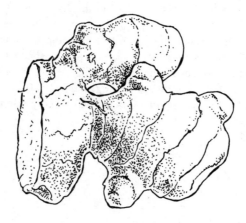

Leeks in Curry Dressing

Serves 4

8 medium leeks, washed and cut into 15-cm (5-6-in) lengths and
cooked until just tender

Dressing
3 tbs corn or sunflower oil
2 tbs wine vinegar
1 tsp curry powder
1 tsp made mustard
salt and freshly ground black pepper
pinch intense sweetener

Arrange the cooled leeks on 4 serving plates. To make the dressing, put all the ingredients in a screw-top jar and shake well. Pour the dressing over the leeks and chill until needed.

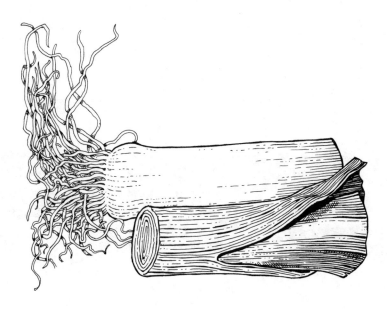

Courgettes à la Grecque

Serves 4

2 tbs olive oil
1 onion, peeled and sliced
1-2 cloves garlic, crushed
450g (1 lb) courgettes, sliced
1 tbs cider vinegar
2 tbs tomato purée
1 tsp thyme
6 tbs water
salt and freshly ground black pepper

Heat the oil in a pan and sauté the onion and garlic for 2-3 minutes. Add the courgettes and cook for 5 minutes, stirring occasionally. Add the vinegar, tomato purée, thyme, water and salt and freshly ground black pepper. Mix all the ingredients together well. Bring them to the boil, cover and simmer for 15 minutes. Serve either hot or cold.

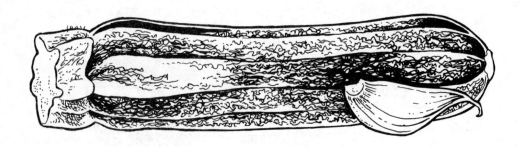

Savoury Crumble

CHO 180g
Kcals 1500

Serves 4-6

2 tsp olive or sunflower oil
1 onion, peeled and chopped
100g (4 oz) mushrooms, sliced
100g (4 oz) carrots, sliced
1 small cauliflower, cut into florets
2 tsp fresh rosemary, chopped
1 tbs wholemeal flour
275ml (½ pt) vegetable stock
salt and freshly ground black pepper
1×425-g (15-oz) can butter beans, drained
1×225-g (8-oz) can kidney beans, drained and refreshed under
cold running water

Topping
50g (2 oz) porridge or jumbo oats
50g (2 oz) 100 per cent wholemeal flour
25g (1 oz) hazelnuts, chopped
25g (1 oz) low-fat spread

Heat the oil in a large frying pan with a close-fitting lid over a moderate heat and fry the onion, mushrooms, carrots and cauliflower. Cover and cook for 5 minutes, stirring frequently. Then, sprinkle the rosemary and flour over the vegetables and cook for 2-3 minutes. Pour on the stock, bring to the boil and simmer gently for 2 minutes. Add salt and freshly ground black pepper to taste, the butter and kidney beans. Pour the mixture into a casserole or ovenproof dish.

For the topping, mix together the oats, flour, hazelnuts and low-fat spread. Sprinkle it on top of the vegetables and bake at 350°F/180°C (Gas Mark 4) for 30 minutes. Serve hot.

Vegetarian Dishes

Stuffed Pepper

Serves 1

1 medium green or red pepper
2 tsp corn or sunflower oil
50g (2 oz) lean bacon, chopped
25g (1 oz) brown rice, cooked
1 tbs frozen peas or sweetcorn
1 tbs raisins
salt and freshly ground black pepper

Slice the top off the pepper and remove the seeds and any white pith. Put the pepper in a saucepan of water and bring to the boil. Simmer for 10 minutes or until it is tender. Drain and keep it warm. Heat the oil in a saucepan and fry the bacon. When it is crisp, add the rice, vegetables and raisins and season to taste with salt and freshly ground black pepper. Heat thoroughly, spoon the mixture into the pepper and serve.

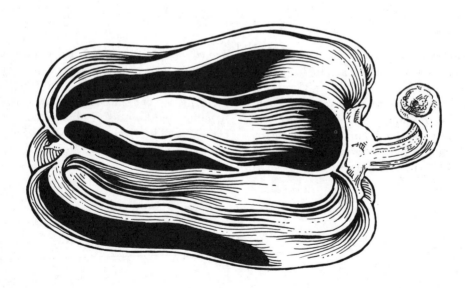

Mushrooms à la Grecque

Serves 4

2 tbs olive oil
1 onion, peeled and chopped
1 clove garlic, crushed
4 tomatoes, skinned, seeded and finely chopped
450g (1 lb) button mushrooms, chopped
1 tbs tomato purée
1 wineglass dry white wine
2 tbs fresh parsley, chopped
salt and freshly ground black pepper

Heat the oil in a pan, add the onion and garlic and fry for 5 minutes. Then add the tomatoes and mushrooms and cook for 5 more minutes, stirring occasionally.

Stir in the tomato purée and wine. Bring to the boil then remove the pan from the heat immediately. Add all but 1 tbs of the parsley and season, stir well and leave the mixture to cool. Chill for at least 2 hours before serving. Top with the reserved parsley before serving.

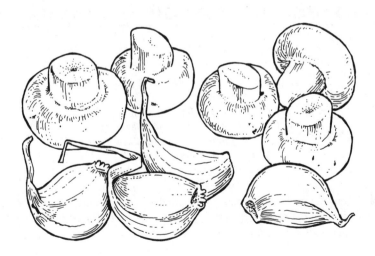

Vegetarian Dishes

Summer Vegetable Salad

Serves 6

2 carrots, sliced
100g (4 oz) broccoli, cooked *al dente*
100g (4 oz) French beans, cooked *al dente*
100g (4 oz) sweetcorn, cooked
50g (2 oz) lentils, cooked
2 courgettes, thinly sliced

Dressing
6 tbs reduced-calorie mayonnaise
bunch tarragon, chopped
2 tbs lemon juice
salt and freshly ground black pepper

Put all the vegetables into a salad bowl.

Mix all the dressing ingredients together then stir it in with the vegetables until they are evenly coated with it. Adjust the seasoning to taste if necessary and chill until needed.

Cheese and Fruit Cocktail

CHO neg
Kcals 260

Serves 4

2 red-skinned dessert apples, chopped (skins left on)
2 sticks celery, chopped
50g (2 oz) reduced-fat cheese, diced
50g (2 oz) grapes, halved and deseeded
grated zest and juice of 1 orange
2 tbs low-fat natural yogurt
a few lettuce leaves, shredded

Put the apples, celery, cheese and grapes into a bowl. Mix the orange juice and yogurt together and add this to the bowl, mixing it together well with the fruit, vegetable and cheese. Arrange the salad on a bed of lettuce and chill until you are ready to serve.

Nut Roast

Makes 6 slices

1 onion, peeled and finely chopped
25g (1 oz) low-fat spread
225g (8 oz) mixed nuts, chopped
100g (4 oz) wholemeal breadcrumbs
275ml (½ pt) vegetable stock
2 tsp yeast extract
pinch of mixed herbs
salt and freshly ground black pepper
slices of tomato to garnish

Sauté the onions until transparent in the low-fat spread that you have melted in a pan. In a large bowl, combine all the other ingredients (reserving 1 tbs of the breadcrumbs) and mix together well. The mixture should be loose. Turn the mixture into a lightly greased 450g (1 lb) loaf tin and sprinkle the reserved breadcrumbs over the top. Bake the loaf at 350°F/180°C (Gas Mark 4) for 30 minutes or until it is golden brown. Allow it to cool before you turn it out, then garnish it with the sliced tomatoes.

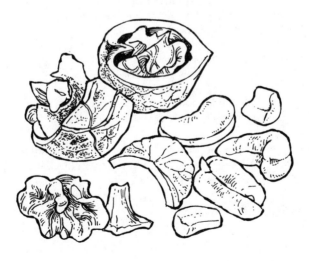

Basic Pancake Mixture

CHO 130g
Kcals 800

Makes 12

150g (5 oz) plain flour
pinch salt
2 × size 3 eggs, lightly beaten
275ml (½ pt) skimmed milk
150ml (¼ pt) water
1 tsp corn or sunflower oil

Sift the flour into a bowl and add a pinch of salt. Make a well in the centre and pour in the eggs. Gradually add the milk and water to the well, stirring round the edge of the well until all the flour becomes amalgamated and smooth. Then mix in the oil and leave to stand for 2-3 hours.

When the batter has stood for this time, lightly grease and heat a heavy-bottomed frying pan. Cook approximately 1 tbs of the mixture at a time, spreading it over the pan. Loosen the edges of the pancakes from the pan before tossing. Allow them to cook for 1 minute on each side.

Fillings

Ratatouille Filling

CHO neg
Kcals 280

1 × 400-g (14-oz) tin chopped tomatoes
2 onions, peeled and chopped
1 small courgette, sliced
1 green pepper, deseeded and sliced
1-2 cloves garlic, crushed
pinch mixed herbs
salt and freshly ground black pepper
50g (2 oz) reduced-fat cheddar cheese, grated

Put all the ingredients except the cheese in a saucepan and simmer for 10-15 minutes, seasoning to taste with salt and freshly ground black pepper.

Fill the pancakes with the ratatouille — putting 2-3 tbs of it in the middle of each pancake — then roll them up and put them in an ovenproof dish. Sprinkle the cheese over them and bake for 10 minutes at 350°F/180°C (Gas Mark 4).

Sweetcorn and Mushroom Filling

25g (1 oz) low-fat spread
225g (8 oz) mushrooms, sliced
1×300-g (11-oz) tin sweetcorn, drained

Cheese sauce
25g (1 oz) low-fat spread
25g (1 oz) flour
275ml (½ pt) skimmed milk
salt and freshly ground black pepper
25g (1 oz) reduced-fat cheddar cheese, grated
salt and freshly ground black pepper

Melt the low-fat spread in a pan, lightly sauté the mushrooms.

Meanwhile, make the cheese sauce. Melt the low-fat spread in a pan, stir in the flour and cook for 1 minute. Then lower the heat and gradually add the milk, stirring all the time. Bring the sauce to a boil and stir quickly until the sauce thickens. Add the cheese and stir until it has melted, then add the mushrooms and sweetcorn. Season to taste with salt and freshly ground black pepper. Use to fill the pancakes in the same way as for the Ratatouille filling.

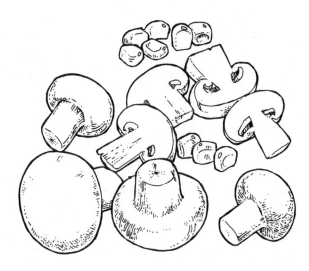

Salads and side dishes

Accompaniments to the main course provide colour, texture and a tasty diversion. By using low-fat, high-fibre ingredients, the selection of appetizing recipes in this section give you all of these and more — health-promoting delicious morsels. Try them on their own, too, for lunches or snacks.

Wholewheat Pasta Salad

CHO 40g
Kcals 440

Serves 2

50g (2 oz) wholewheat pasta, cooked
1 medium or 2 small carrots, sliced
½ green pepper, deseeded and cut into strips
2 stalks celery, chopped
½ tsp garlic powder
1 tbs Worcestershire or soy sauce
fresh parsley, chopped, to garnish

Mix all the ingredients, except the parsley, together in a bowl. Garnish the salad with the chopped parsley.

Waldorf Salad

CHO 60g
Kcals 570

Serves 4-6

3 red apples, diced
2 tbs lemon juice
50g (2 oz) walnuts, chopped
1 head of celery, chopped
300g (10 fl oz) low-fat natural yogurt
a few lettuce leaves to garnish

Put all but a third of the apple in a bowl and drizzle the lemon juice over to prevent it browning. Mix the nuts, celery and natural yogurt with the apple. Arrange the lettuce leaves and salad on a serving dish. Use the reserved apple to garnish the salad.

Italian Bean Salad

CHO 50g
Kcals 670

Serves 4

1×425-g (15-oz) tin cannellini beans, drained
1×200-g (7-oz) tin tuna in brine, drained
1 small onion, peeled and sliced
4 tbs Mustard Dressing recipe (see page 132)

Put all the ingredients into a bowl and toss together until they are well mixed. Chill in the refrigerator before serving.

Red Kidney Beans with Walnuts

CHO 30g
Kcals 800

Serves 4

1×225-g (8-oz) tin red kidney beans, drained and refreshed under
cold running water
1 small fennel bulb, finely chopped
1 onion, peeled and sliced
50g (2 oz) walnuts, chopped
3 tbs olive oil
2-3 tbs fresh parsley, chopped
2 cloves garlic, crushed
salt and freshly ground black pepper

Mix the kidney beans, fennel, onion and walnuts together in a salad bowl. Season the olive oil with the parsley, garlic and salt and freshly ground black pepper. Dress the vegetable mixture with it and leave to marinate for an hour or so before serving.

Autumn Salad

CHO 40g
Kcals 680

Serves 6

1 crispy lettuce, shredded
1 green pepper, deseeded and sliced
2 courgettes, thinly sliced
75g (3 oz) green lentils, cooked
1×Low-calorie French Dressing recipe (see page 131)
salt and freshly ground black pepper
1 tsp ground cumin
50g (2 oz) unsalted peanuts, chopped and toasted

Put the lettuce and green pepper into a salad bowl. Add the courgettes and lentils. Pour the Low-calorie French Dressing over the salad and mix so it coats all the ingredients well. Season to taste with salt and freshly ground black pepper. Just before serving, toss in the chopped peanuts.

Rice Salad

CHO 145g
Kcals 1095

Serves 6

175g (6 oz) brown rice, cooked
225g (8 oz) tomatoes, chopped
1 green pepper, deseeded and sliced
10 green olives, stoned and halved
50g (2 oz) unsalted peanuts, chopped and toasted
1×Low-calorie French Dressing recipe (see page 131)
salt and freshly ground black pepper

Put the rice into a bowl. Add the tomatoes, pepper, olives and peanuts and mix everything together well. Pour in the Low-calorie French Dressing and season to taste with salt and freshly ground black pepper. Chill until you are ready to serve.

Fruit and Vegetable Mixed Salad

CHO 100g
Kcals 550

Serves 6-8

3 carrots, peeled and coarsely grated
2 apples, cored and sliced
2 pears, cored and sliced
6 celery sticks, finely sliced
1 green pepper, deseeded and sliced
½ cucumber, diced
50g (2 oz) raisins
1 tsp lemon juice
salt and freshly ground black pepper
1×150-g (5-fl oz) carton low-fat natural yogurt

Put all the prepared fruit and vegetables into a bowl. Add the lemon juice and seasonings to the yogurt. Mix the yogurt dressing with the salad ingredients and chill well before serving.

Low-calorie French Dressing

CHO neg
Kcals 100

Makes 100ml/4 fl oz

6 tbs cider or wine vinegar
1 tbs olive oil
½ tsp dry mustard
salt and freshly ground black pepper

Measure all the ingredients into a jar with a screw-top lid. Shake them together well and store in the refrigerator until the dressing is needed. Shake the jar vigorously before using as the ingredients settle.
Note This recipe will keep for 2-3 days in the refrigerator.

Salads and side dishes

Mustard Dressing

CHO neg
Kcals 330

Makes 100ml/4 fl oz

3 tbs olive oil
2 tbs cider vinegar
1 tsp wholegrain mustard
1 small onion, peeled and grated
1 clove garlic, crushed
pinch intense sweetener
salt and freshly ground black pepper

Measure all the ingredients into a screw-top jar and shake it well until the ingredients are well mixed. Chill the dressing in the refrigerator until you need it. Shake the jar well before serving to remix the ingredients as they tend to settle after the initial making.

Note This recipe will keep for 2-3 days in the refrigerator.

Tsatziki

CHO 20g
Kcals 160

Serves 4-6

2×150-g (5-fl oz) cartons low-fat natural yogurt
10-cm (4-in) piece cucumber, diced
1 tbs fresh mint, chopped
1 clove garlic, crushed (optional)
1 sprig fresh mint to garnish

Mix all the ingredients together and chill it well before you serve it. Garnish the Tzatziki with the sprig of mint.

Potato and Sprout Bake

CHO 80g
Kcals 550

Serves 4-6

450g (1 lb) potatoes, peeled and diced
225g (8 oz) Brussels sprouts, peeled and trimmed
15g (½ oz) low-fat spread
freshly grated nutmeg
salt and freshly ground black pepper
25g (1 oz) reduced-fat cheddar cheese, grated

Cook the potatoes and sprouts in boiling water for about 15 minutes. Drain, then mash them together with the low-fat spread, nutmeg and season with salt and freshly ground black pepper. Spoon the mixture into a heatproof dish, sprinkle the cheese over the top and grill until the cheese is bubbling and golden brown. Serve immediately.

Cooked Chicory

CHO neg
Kcals 240

Serves 4

50g (2 oz) low-fat spread
450g (1 lb) chicory, leaves separated from the stem
pinch salt
pinch intense sweetener
juice of 1 lemon

Melt the low-fat spread in a pan and toss the chicory leaves in it. Add the salt, sweetener and lemon juice and cover. Cook over a gentle heat for 10 minutes, then serve immediately.

Salads and side dishes

Braised Celery

Serves 4

1 onion, peeled and chopped
1 medium carrot, peeled and chopped
1 clove garlic, crushed
25g (1 oz) low-fat spread
2 small heads of celery, split into individual sticks
150ml (¼ pt) vegetable stock
salt and freshly ground black pepper
1-2 tbs fresh parsley, chopped

Lightly sauté the onion, carrot and garlic in the low-fat spread in a pan for 5 minutes. Transfer the vegetables to an ovenproof casserole. Put the celery on top of the vegetables. Pour the stock over it and season well with salt and freshly ground black pepper. Cover and bake at 350°F/180°C (Gas Mark 4) for approximately 1-1½ hours, turning the celery occasionally in the juices. Serve this dish hot, with the parsley sprinkled over it just before serving.

Spring Cabbage

Serves 4

25g (1 oz) low-fat spread
675g (1½ lb) spring cabbage, shredded
1 onion, peeled and chopped
2 rashers, streaky bacon, rind removed and chopped
pinch grated nutmeg

Heat the low-fat spread in a large saucepan, add all the ingredients, cover and cook very gently for 20-30 minutes, until the cabbage is just tender, stirring frequently. Serve immediately.

Puddings and desserts

There is no doubt that everyone loves a good pudding or sophisticated dessert, whether it is hot or cold. What could be a better ending to a meal than a slice of cheesecake or a hearty crumble?

The recipes that follow use fruits that are high in fibre and a good source of vitamins, together with other high-fibre ingredients, such as wholemeal flour and dried fruits, and low-fat ingredients, such as low-fat spreads and dairy products. Where possible the virtually calorie-free artificial sweeteners are used instead of sugar to sweeten a dish and where sugar is used, the quantities have been reduced as much as possible. All this means that you can eat a lovely dessert without feeling guilty — as long as you don't get too carried away!

Eve's Pudding

Serves 8-10

450g (1 lb) cooking apples, peeled, cored and sliced
zest and juice of 1 orange and 1 lemon
25g (1 oz) hazelnuts, finely chopped
2 tbs water

Topping
100g (4 oz) low-fat spread
50g (2 oz) caster sugar
2 × size 3 eggs, beaten
100g (4 oz) wholemeal self-raising flour
pinch baking powder
pinch cinnamon
1 tbs boiling water

Put the sliced apples in a deep 20 by 25-cm (8 by 10-in) baking dish. Add the zest and juice of the orange and lemon, the nuts and water and mix them together well. Cover with foil and bake in the oven at 375°F/190°C (Gas Mark 5) for 10-12 minutes.

Meanwhile, make the topping. Cream the low-fat spread and sugar together until the texture is light and fluffy. Add the beaten eggs gradually, beating the mixture well between each addition. Gradually add the flour, folding it into the creamed mixture. Add the baking powder, cinnamon and water and mix them into the mixture. Spread the topping evenly over the fruit and return the dish to the oven for a further 25-30 minutes, or until the topping is well risen and springs back when touched. The pudding may be served hot or cold.

Baked Apples

CHO 50g
Kcals 190

Serves 2

2 medium cooking apples, cores removed
25g (1 oz) raisins
½ tsp ground cinnamon
½ tsp ground mixed spice

Slit the apple skins from top to bottom at intervals and then put them in an ovenproof dish. Mix the raisins with the spices and fill the core of each apple with the fruit mixture. Cover the dish with foil and bake at 350°F/180°C (Gas Mark 4) for about 30-40 minutes.

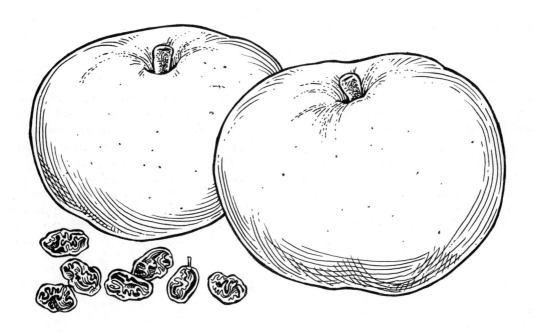

Bakewell Tart

Makes 8-10 portions

Pastry
75g (3 oz) wholemeal flour
25g (1 oz) plain flour
pinch salt
25g (1 oz) low-fat spread
25g (1 oz) white polyunsaturated vegetable fat
cold water to mix

Filling
2 tbs pure fruit spread
50g (2 oz) low-fat spread
25g (1 oz) caster sugar
50g (2 oz) ground rice
25g (1 oz) ground almonds
1×size 3 egg, beaten
few drops almond essence (optional)
blanched almonds to decorate

Make the pastry by sieving the two flours and salt together into a bowl, cutting in the fats until they are well mixed with the flour and then stirring in a little cold water at a time until the mixture forms a smooth, pliable dough, neither too hard nor too soft. Line an 18-cm (7-in) fluted flan ring with the pastry, saving the oddments left over. Spread the pure fruit spread over the bottom.

Now make the filling. Cream the low-fat spread and sugar until the mixture becomes light and fluffy. Mix together the ground rice and ground almonds and add this to the creamed mixture with the beaten egg and almond essence (if using), combining all the ingredients together well. Spread the mixture over the jam. Knead the reserved scraps of pastry together, roll it out and cut it into strips. Decorate the top of the tart by making a lattice pattern with the strips and dotting with blanched almonds. Bake the tart at 375°F/190°C (Gas Mark 5) for 30-35 minutes.

Peach Pudding

Serves 10

75g (3 oz) low-fat spread
50g (2 oz) caster sugar
2×size 3 eggs, beaten
50g (2 oz) wholemeal self-raising flour
25g (1 oz) ground almonds
1 tsp ground cinnamon
3 fresh peaches, peeled, stoned and sliced
2 tsp demerara sugar

Cream the low-fat spread and sugar until the mixture has become pale. Beat in the eggs a little at a time alternately with the flour, ground almonds and half the cinnamon. Spoon the mixture into a lightly greased 23-cm (9-in) round, shallow ovenproof dish or pie plate. Arrange the peach slices over the mixture and push them into it.

Mix the remaining cinnamon with the demerara sugar and sprinkle it over the pudding, then bake it at 375°F/190°C (Gas Mark 5) for approximately 30 minutes or until it has cooked. The mixture should have risen, be golden brown and the sugar should have caramelized.

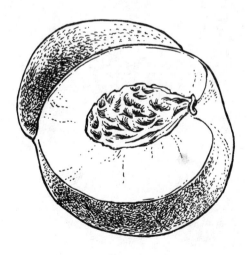

Puddings and desserts

Trifle

Serves 6

1×425-g (15-oz) tin fruit cocktail in natural juice
1 packet sugar-free jelly crystals
2 tbs custard powder
275ml (½ pt) skimmed milk
intense artificial sweetener to taste *(granulated if poss.)*
5 fl. oz. 150ml (¼ pt) whipping cream, whipped
a few flaked almonds, toasted

Drain the fruit and reserve the juice. Arrange the fruit in the bottom of a bowl. Make up the jelly crystals according to the directions on the packet and make up to 550ml (1 pt) using the reserved fruit juice. Pour the jelly onto the fruit and leave to set. Make the custard according to the directions on the tin and sweeten if necessary. Pour it over the fruit and top with the whipped cream and toasted almonds. Chill the trifle well before serving.

Put whipped cream around edge in rosettes.

Shortly before serving, strew the toasted almonds over the custard.

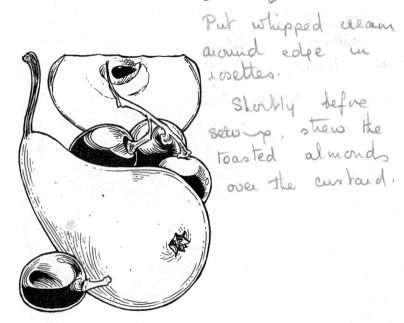

Prune Flan

CHO 190g
Kcals 1680

Serves 6-8

200-g (7-oz) tin prunes in fruit juice, drained and the juice reserved

Pastry
100g (4 oz) wholemeal flour
50g (2 oz) plain flour
50g (2 oz) low-fat spread
25g (1 oz) white polyunsaturated vegetable fat
25g (1 oz) ground almonds
cold water to bind

Custard
1 tbs custard powder
150ml (¼ pt) skimmed milk
intense artificial sweetener to taste

Almond filling
50g (2 oz) ground almonds
1 tsp intense artificial sweetener
2 tbs water

Make the pastry by rubbing the fat into the flour until it resembles fine breadcrumbs. Stir in the ground almonds and bind with a little cold water. Chill the pastry for 30 minutes before use.

Meanwhile, make the custard. Blend the custard powder with 1 tbs of the milk and warm the rest of the milk. Whisk in the custard powder mixture until it is well mixed. Heat the custard gently, stirring, until it has thickened and sweeten to taste.

Roll out pastry and line an 18-cm (7-in) flan ring. Bake it blind at 350°F/190°C (Gas Mark 4) for 10-12 minutes.

To make the almond filling, mix the almonds and sweetener and stir in sufficient water to bind them together.

Cut each prune down one side and remove the stone. Then fill each prune with the almond mixture, spoon the custard into the cooled flan case and arrange the filled prunes on top. Brush the flan with the reserved prune juice to glaze. Leave it to cool and then chill it until just before serving.

Puddings and desserts

Raspberry and Kiwi Whip

CHO 30g
Kcals 280

Serves 4-6

100g (4 oz) quark or skimmed milk cheese
1×150-g (5-fl oz) carton low-fat natural yogurt
225g (8 oz) raspberries, fresh or frozen, puréed
intense artificial sweetener to taste
2 kiwi fruit, peeled and sliced

Mix the soft cheese and yogurt together in a bowl. Add the raspberry purée and sweetener to taste. Arrange the kiwi fruit in individual dishes or 1 large bowl, reserving 2 or 3 slices. Pour the raspberry mixture over the fruit and chill in a refrigerator before serving. Then decorate with the reserved kiwi fruit slices.

Yogurt Gooseberry Fool

CHO 10g
Kcals 160

Serves 6

450g (1 lb) gooseberries, topped and tailed
intense artificial sweetener to taste
1×150-g (5-fl oz) carton low-fat natural yogurt or diet gooseberry yogurt
1-2 drops green food colouring (optional)

Put the gooseberries in a pan with a little water and cook them gently until the fruit is soft. Purée the gooseberries in a blender and press through a sieve to remove the seeds. Fold the yogurt into the fruit purée. Add 1-2 drops of green food colouring if using. Divide the fool between 6 individual glass dessert bowl or wine goblets and chill until you are ready to serve.

Note Because each portion will have an insignificant amount of CHO, it does not have to be counted in the diet.

Fruit Yogurt Whips

CHO 60g
Kcals 410

Serves 4

1 banana, peeled and chopped
1 tsp lemon juice
2×size 3 egg whites
1 tbs intense artificial sweetener
2×150-g (5-fl oz) cartons low-fat natural yogurt
25g (1 oz) dried mixed fruit
25g (1 oz) chopped hazelnuts

Mix the banana with the lemon juice in a bowl to prevent it browning. Whisk the egg whites until they are stiff, then gently fold in the sweetener and yogurt using a metal spoon. Fold in the dried fruit and nuts, reserving a little to decorate the whips. Divide the mixture between 4 dishes and sprinkle each one with the reserved nuts. Serve immediately.

Variation
Try using a diet fruit-flavoured yogurt instead of the natural yogurt, say, apple and cinnamon, peach or apricot.

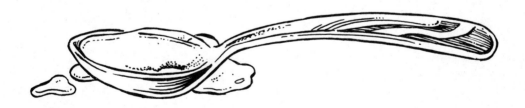

Puddings and desserts

Yogurt Snow with Raspberry Sauce

CHO 20g
Kcals 160

Serves 3-4

225-g (8-fl oz) low-fat natural yogurt
intense artificial sweetener to taste
1 egg white, beaten until stiff

Raspberry sauce
100g (4 oz) raspberries
juice of 1 lemon
intense artificial sweetener to taste
a few mint leaves to decorate

Drain the yogurt in a muslin-lined sieve for several hours (preferably overnight). Add the sweetener to the drained yogurt and fold in the beaten egg white. Spoon the Snow into ramekin dishes and chill for about an hour.

Meanwhile, purée the raspberries — reserving 3 or 4 to decorate — in a liquidizer for several minutes. Add the lemon juice and sweetener and purée again. Strain the sauce into a serving jug. Decorate the Snow with the reserved raspberries and the mint leaves and serve the sauce in a jug for people to help themselves.

COOK'S TIP
You can use a clean 'all-purpose cloth' if you don't happen to have any muslin.

Apple Delight

Serves 2

2×150-g (5-fl oz) cartons low-fat natural yogurt
2 eating apples, peeled, cored and grated
zest and juice of ½ lemon
intense artificial sweetener to taste (optional)
2 walnut halves to decorate

Pour the yogurt into a bowl. Add the apple, lemon zest and juice and sweeten to taste. Pour the Delight into 2 individual dishes and chill well before serving. Top each dish with a walnut half and serve.

Raspberry Mousse

Serves 6-8

1 sachet raspberry sugar-free jelly crystals
1×400-g (14-oz) tin raspberries in juice
2×size 3 egg whites
1×150-ml (5-fl oz) carton whipping cream

Make the jelly up to 275ml (½ pt) with boiling water. Purée the raspberries and make up to 275ml (½ pt) with water (sieve it to remove the pips if you prefer a smooth texture). Add the raspberry mixture to the jelly and, once it has cooled, put it in the refrigerator until it has nearly set — until the jelly coats the back of a spoon (this usually takes about 1 hour). Whisk the cream until it is thick and stir it into the jelly mixture. Beat the egg whites until they are stiff and gently fold them into the jelly using a metal spoon. Then pour the mousse into a dish and leave it to set in the refrigerator.

Note An individual/single serving would have a negligible amount of CHO.

Marbled Apricots

Serves 4-6

450g (1 lb) fresh apricots, cut in half and the stones removed
200g (7 oz) fat-free fromage frais
intense artificial sweetener to taste (optional)

Stew the apricots in a little water until they are tender. Leave them to cool then purée them in a blender or food processor.

Pour the fromage frais into a 500-ml/1-pt glass bowl, add the sweetener, if using, spoon in the apricot purée and blend only until a marble effect occurs — do not mix them together thoroughly. Chill the mixture before serving.

Baked Figs

Serves 6

6 fresh figs, stalks removed
2 tbs apricot pure fruit spread
grated zest and juice of 1 orange
1×150-g (5-fl oz) carton low-fat natural yogurt

Make 2 cuts in the top of each fig, about three quarters of the way through, to divide the figs into quarters. Squeeze the base of each fig, opening it out into a flower shape to reveal the flesh and seeds inside.

Put 1 tsp pure fruit spread into each fig and put them in a lightly greased baking dish. Top them with a little orange zest, then spoon the orange juice over. Cover the dish with foil and bake at 375°F/190°C (Gas Mark 5) for 15 minutes, then serve them hot with the yogurt.

Pears Cassis

CHO 70g
Kcals 350

Serves 4

4 pears, peeled, cored and halved
275ml (½ pt) water
1 vanilla pod or 2-3 drops vanilla essence
275-g (10-oz) tin blackcurrants in juice
intense artificial sweetener to taste
2 tsp arrowroot

Put the pear halves in a pan with the water and vanilla. Cover the pan, bring to the boil, then simmer until the pears look almost transparent (this will take about 20-30 minutes).

Meanwhile, purée the blackcurrants.

When the pears are ready, drain them, reserving the cooking liquid, put them in a serving dish and keep them warm. Make the blackcurrant purée up to 425ml/¾ pt with the reserved liquid from the pears, adding sweetener to taste, and heat it gently. Mix the arrowroot with 2 tbs of the pear liquid and add it to the pan, stirring as you do so and until it thickens slightly, then pour it over the pears and serve.

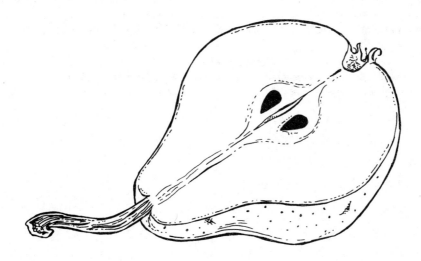

147   **Puddings and desserts**

Cheesecake

Serves 6-8

50g (2 oz) low-fat spread
175g (6 oz) wholemeal shortbread, crushed
1 sachet gelatine
finely grated rind and juice of 1 orange
225g (8 oz) skimmed milk cheese or quark
1×150-g (5-fl oz) carton low-fat natural yogurt
liquid sweetener to taste
2×size 3 eggs, separated
100g (4 oz) fresh or frozen raspberries

Melt the low-fat spread and mix it with the crushed shortbread. Press it down evenly in the bottom of an 18-cm (7-in) spring release or a loose bottomed tin. Leave it to chill in the refrigerator for 30 minutes.

Meanwhile, dissolve gelatine in 3 tbs of hot water. Put the orange rind and juice and skimmed milk cheese or quark into a bowl. Add the yogurt, sweetener and egg yolks and mix them together well. Add the cooled gelatine and mix well. Whisk the egg whites until they are stiff and then lightly fold them into the yogurt mixture. Carefully pour the mixture into the tin, smooth the top and chill for several hours, preferably overnight.

Remove the cheesecake from the tin, leaving the base in place, and put it on a flat serving plate. Decorate the top with the raspberries.

COOK'S TIP:
You can freeze the cheesecake if you wish, but do so before putting the fruit on top and decorate it instead when you defrost it to use at a later date.

Fresh Fruit Jelly

CHO 40g
Kcals 190

Serves 6-8

1 packet sugar-free jelly crystals
1 red apple, cored and sliced
1 orange, peeled and segmented
20 grapes (10 black and 10 white)
You can use any fresh fruit you like that is in season.
Strawberries, bananas, tangerines and white grapes
are all good alternatives.

Make up the jelly crystals according to the directions on the packet. Put the fruit into a bowl and pour the jelly over it. Leave it to cool then chill it until it has set in a refrigerator before serving.

Peach Ice-cream

CHO 80g
Kcals 560

Serves 6-8

1×425-g (15-oz) tin peach slices in juice
1×150-g (5-fl oz) carton low-fat natural yogurt
1×170-g (6-7-oz) tin evaporated milk, well chilled

Put the peaches and the juice into a blender or food processor and blend for 1-2 minutes. Whisk the evaporated milk until it is thick and has doubled in volume. Whisk in the yogurt and gently fold the peach purée into the mixture. Pour it into a freezer-proof container and freeze it until it has frozen around the edges (this takes about 1-2 hours). Beat the mixture breaking up the crystals and pour it back into the container or individual cartons and freeze it uncovered.

Put the ice-cream in a refrigerator for 10-15 minutes to soften a little before you serve it.

Puddings and desserts

Fruit Fool

CHO 50g
Kcals 280

Serves 2

175g (6 oz) blackcurrants
4 tsp custard powder
150ml (¼ pt) skimmed milk
1×150-g (5-fl oz) carton low-fat natural yogurt
1 tsp intense artificial sweetener

Cook the blackcurrants in approximately 2 tbs water until they are soft, then sieve or liquidize the fruit.

Make the custard by mixing the custard powder with 4 tsp of the milk, warming the rest of the milk, mixing in the custard powder mixture and stirring continuously until it thickens, then take it off the heat and leave it to cool.

When the custard has cooled, add the puréed fruit and yogurt to the custard and mix them together thoroughly. Sweeten the fool to taste and chill before serving.

Grape Jelly

CHO 30g
Kcals 190

Serves 6

150ml (¼ pt) unsweetened white grape juice
generous 3 tbs lemon juice
275ml (½ pt) water
15g (½ oz) gelatine, dissolved in 3 tbs cold water
artificial sweetener to taste
75g (3 oz) small black or green grapes, halved and depipped

Pour the grape and lemon juice and water into a dish. Add the dissolved gelatine, stirring, then chill the jelly until the mixture has the consistency of unbeaten egg white. Then stir in the grapes and chill until the jelly has set.

Pears in Mulled Wine

Serves 4

4 ripe even-sized pears
275ml (½ pt) red wine
pinch of grated nutmeg
1 stick cinnamon
rind of half a lemon
few drops lemon juice
4 cloves
intense artificial sweetener to taste

Peel the pears, leaving the stalks on. Slice a sliver off the bottom so that they will stand up. Put all the ingredients, except the pears, into a saucepan and heat them for 5 minutes. Pour everything into a small, deep-sided dish and stand the pears in it, basting them with the wine mixture. Bake the pears at 350°F/180°C (Gas Mark 4) for 30 minutes, basting them occasionally. Serve the pears immediately, with a little of the cooking juices dribbled over them.

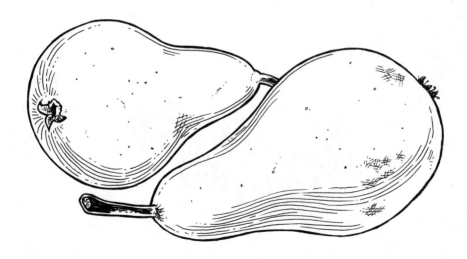

Puddings and desserts

Summer Pudding

Serves 6

675g (1½-2 lb) mixed soft fruits, such as blackcurrants, redcurrants,
raspberries and blackberries
intense artificial sweetener to taste
6 or so slices of stale white bread, crusts removed

Put the soft fruits in a saucepan and cook them gently for 5 minutes or until the juices run and the fruits soften and sweeten to taste.

Meanwhile, line the bottom and sides of a 825ml (1½ pt) pudding basin with the bread, ensuring that there are no gaps between the slices and reserving 1½ slices for the top.

Put the fruit and all but 2 tbs of the juice into the bread-lined basin, cover with the reserved bread. Put a plate over the top and weigh it down with weights or a heavy tin. Chill the pudding overnight.

To unmould the pudding, hold the serving plate, inverted, over the top of the basin and turn the pudding over. Pour the reserved fruit juice over the pudding just before serving.

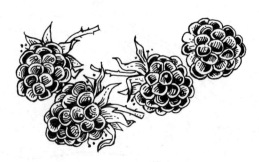

Home baking

Home-baked bread and teatime treats are pleasures that shouldn't be a thing of the past. You can still enjoy them if you like to treat yourself occasionally. They needn't take long to make either and beat bought versions hands down.

The recipes for traditional favourites here have been modified so that high-fibre, low-fat and low-sugar ingredients replace some of the bad-for-you ones *without* sacrificing taste. Try some with your afternoon tea today!

Wholemeal Bread

Makes 3 450-g (1-lb) loaves

900g (2 lb) wholemeal flour
1 tbs salt
50g (2 oz) low-fat spread
1 tbs easy-blend dried yeast
1 tbs malt extract
550ml (1 pt) tepid water

Combine the flour, salt and yeast, then rub in the low-fat spread. Dissolve the yeast and the malt in the water and gradually add it to the flour, mixing it in well. Knead it to a soft dough, then turn it out onto a floured board and knead for 10-15 minutes until it is smooth and elastic. Divide the mixture into 3 and put each in a lightly oiled 450-g (1 lb) loaf tin. Put them in a warm place to prove (double in size).

Bake them at 400°F/200°C (Gas Mark 6) for 10 minutes then reduce the temperature to 350°F/180°C (Gas Mark 4) for 25-35 minutes. You can tell that they are done if when you turn them out they sound hollow when you rap the bottoms. Turn them out of the tins and leave them to cool on a wire rack.

COOK'S TIP:
These loaves freeze well wrapped in foil once they have cooled.

Victoria Sandwich

Serves 8

100g (4 oz) low-fat spread
50g (2 oz) caster sugar
2 × size 3 eggs, lightly beaten
1 tbs hot water
100g (4 oz) self-raising wholemeal flour
pinch baking powder

Cream the low-fat spread and sugar together until the mixture is light and creamy. Beat in the eggs and water. Sieve the flour and baking powder into another bowl, then gradually add it to the creamed mixture, folding it in so that they are thoroughly mixed together.

Divide the mixture between 2 15-cm (6-in), lightly greased sandwich tins and bake at 350°F/180°C (Gas Mark 4) for 20-25 minutes until they have risen well, spring back when touched and are golden brown. Turn them out onto a wire tray to cool.

You can then fill the cake with pure fruit spread and whipped cream and sprinkle a little powdered intense sweetener over the top or fill it with pure fruit spread and some of the Butter Icing recipe on page 168. A pretty finishing touch is to lay a paper doily on top of the filled cake and sift a little powdered sweetener over it. When you lift the doily, there will be a lacy pattern.

Note If you use jam in the cake remember to add the CHO and calories. 1 oz pure fruit spread contains approx. 10g CHO, 35 cals. If using whipped cream a 142ml/5 fl oz carton contains 510 calories.

Fairy Cakes

CHO 90g
Kcals 660

Makes 10

50g (2 oz) low-fat spread
25g (1 oz) caster sugar
1 × size 3 egg, beaten
50g (2 oz) self-raising wholemeal flour
50g (2 oz) raisins
1 tbs boiling water, if needed

Cream the low-fat spread and sugar together until the mixture pales in colour. Add half the beaten egg and 1 tsp of the flour and beat well. Add the remaining egg and 1 tsp of the flour and beat well. Add the remaining flour gradually and the raisins, folding them in gently using a metal spoon. The mixture now should be of a dropping consistency (if it is not, add the 1 tbs of boiling water).

Spoon equal amounts of the mixture into 10 paper cases in a patty tin and bake on the middle shelf of the oven for 10-15 minutes at 350°F/180°C (Gas Mark 4) until the Fairy Cakes have risen well, are golden brown and firm to the touch.

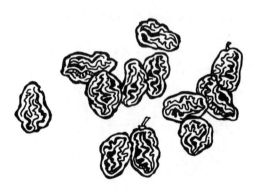

Butterfly Cakes

Makes 12-15

1×Victoria Sandwich recipe (see page 155)
a little granular intense artificial sweetener
Butter Icing recipe (see page 168) flavoured with 1-2 drops vanilla
essence

Prepare the Victoria Sandwich recipe as given on page 155 and divide the mixture between 12-15 paper cases in patty tins. Bake them in a 350°F/180°C (Gas Mark 4) oven for 12-15 minutes until the Cakes have risen and are golden brown. Remove them from the tin and leave them to cool on a wire rack.

Meanwhile, prepare the Butter Icing as given on page 168.

When the Cakes have cooled, cut a slice from the top of each bun and put a tsp of the Butter Icing over the cut cake. Cut the removed slices in half and replace them on the cakes, angling them into the Butter Icing to form 'wings'. Dust the Cakes with granular intense artificial sweetener. The cakes are tastiest when they are fresh.

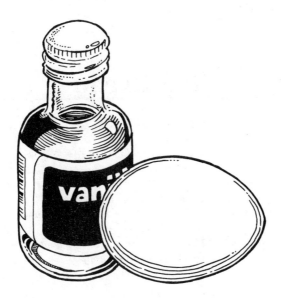

Banana and Walnut Slices

CHO 160g
Kcals 1580

Makes 16

100g (4 oz) low-fat spread
50g (2 oz) sugar
2×size 3 eggs
100g (4 oz) wholemeal self-raising flour
1 tsp baking powder
2 small bananas, mashed
75g (3 oz) walnuts, chopped

Preheat the oven to 375°F/190°C (Gas Mark 5).

Cream the low-fat spread and the sugar together until the mixture is light and fluffy. Beat in the eggs, one at a time, adding a tbs of the flour with the second egg. Fold in the remaining flour and the baking powder together with the bananas.

Spread the mixture evenly in a lined and greased 15 by 25-cm (6 by 10-in) shallow tin and sprinkle the walnuts over the top. Bake in the preheated oven for 20-25 minutes.

When the mixture has cooked, leave it in the tin but cut it into 16 equal pieces. Leave the tin on a wire rack to cool, then turn the slices out and store them in an airtight container.

Tea Bread

CHO 210g
Kcals 1680

Makes 1 450-g (1-lb) loaf

100g (4 oz) low-fat spread
50g (2 oz) caster sugar
1×size 3 egg, beaten
2 small bananas, mashed
1×150-g (5-fl oz) carton low-fat natural yogurt
50g (2 oz) white self-raising flour
100g (4 oz) wholemeal self-raising flour
50g (2 oz) walnuts, chopped
25g (1 oz) sultanas

Cream the low-fat spread and sugar until the mixture is light and fluffy. Add the egg and beat it in well. Stir in the bananas and yogurt. Gently fold in the flour, walnuts and sultanas.

Spoon the mixture into a lightly greased 450-g (1-lb) loaf tin and bake at 375°F/190°C (Gas Mark 5) for approximately 1 hour or until it is cooked (check it by inserting a clean skewer into the centre and leaving it there for a couple of seconds — if it comes out clean, the Tea Bread is done).

Rhubarb and Raisin Cake

CHO 210g
Kcals 1260

This cake freezes well. Just wrap it in foil once it has cooled.

Makes 12 portions

225g (8 oz) rhubarb, chopped
50g (2 oz) low-fat spread
225g (8 oz) self-raising wholemeal flour
1 tsp baking powder
100g (4 oz) raisins
1 × size 3 egg, beaten
4 tbs skimmed milk

Cook the rhubarb in a little water for 5-10 minutes. Rub the low-fat spread into the flour and baking powder, which you have sieved together into a bowl. Add the rhubarb and raisins and mix them in. Add the egg and milk and mix them in well. Pour the mixture into a lightly oiled 18-cm (7-in) cake tin and bake at 375°F/190°C (Gas Mark 5) for 1 hour. Turn the cake out and leave it to cool on a wire rack.

Home baking

Celebration Cake 1,

**CHO 320g
Kcals 2300**

This cake freezes well wrapped in foil.

Makes 24 portions

see Xmas cake P. 176

25g (1 oz) sugar
75g (3 oz) sultanas
75g (3 oz) currants
75g (3 oz) raisins   *seedless*
300ml (½ pt) Guinness
50g (2 oz) low-fat spread
225g (8 oz) 100 per cent wholemeal flour   *(Try ¼ cornflour ?*
½ tsp baking powder   *¾ plain)*
1 tsp mixed spice
75g (3 oz) walnuts, chopped
3 × size 3 eggs, beaten

Put the sugar, fruit and Guinness in a pan, bring it to the boil, then leave it to simmer for 20 minutes. Add the low-fat spread and leave it to cool. Add the beaten egg to the mixture. Sieve the flour and baking powder together into a bowl, then stir it into the pan. Pour the mixture into a well-oiled 18-cm (7-in) square tin and bake at

350°F/180°C (Gas Mark 4) for 1-1½ hours. Leave it to cool in the tin on a wire rack.

To test whether the Cake is done, insert a clean skewer into the centre and leave it there for 2 seconds. If the skewer is clean when you pull it out, the cake is done.

or 8" round

Keep to traditional method:
a) sift flour & spices & baking powder
b) mix fruit & nuts
c) cream fat & sugar separately.
d) gradually beat in eggs & flour. alternately add remaining flour, fruit & 'booze'

Try slower cooking 4 hrs. at '1'

Date and Walnut Loaf

CHO 370g
Kcals 2290

Makes 1 900-g (2-lb) loaf

225g (8 oz) stoned dates, chopped
½ tsp bicarbonate of soda
½ tsp salt
150ml (¼ pt) boiling water
100g (4 oz) low-fat spread
75g (3 oz) brown sugar
1×size 3 egg, beaten
225g (8 oz) wholemeal self-raising flour
50g (2 oz) walnuts, chopped

Put the dates, bicarbonate of soda and salt in a basin, pour over the boiling water over them and put to one side.

Meanwhile, cream the low-fat spread and sugar and beat in the egg. Stir in flour, nuts and date mixture and stir until all the ingredients are combined. Pour the mixture into a lightly greased 900-g (2-lb) loaf tin and bake at 350°F/180°C (Gas Mark 4) for 1-1½ hours. To test whether the Loaf is done, poke a clean skewer into the centre of it, leave it there for 2 seconds, then if it comes out clean, it is done.

Then turn it out onto a wire rack and leave it to cool. When it has cooled, store in an airtight container.

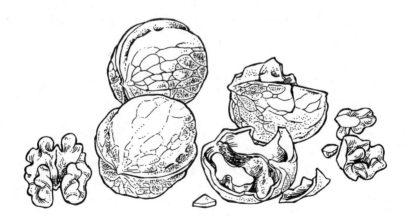

Home baking

Prune and Nut Cake

CHO 190g
Kcals 1310

Makes 12 portions

225g (8 oz) self-raising wholemeal flour
pinch salt
1 tsp grated nutmeg
pinch ground all spice
grated zest of 1 small orange
25g (1 oz) low-fat spread
50g (2 oz) walnuts, chopped
75g (3 oz) stoneless prunes, chopped
1×size 3 egg, beaten
100ml (3 fl oz) skimmed milk
3 tbs juice from the orange

Sieve the flour, salt and spices into a bowl and add the orange zest. Mix in the low-fat spread using a fork. Stir in the walnuts and prunes and beat in the egg, milk and orange juice until everything is well mixed. Turn the mixture into a greased 15-cm (6-in) round cake tin and bake at 375°F/190°C (Gas Mark 5) for 40-45 minutes or until the Cake is well risen and golden brown and a skewer pierced through the centre of the cake comes out clean. Allow it to cool before serving.

COOK'S TIP:

Serve this with Curd Cheese Topping (see page 168) for a special occasion.

Rock Cakes

Makes 14

100g (4 oz) self-raising wholemeal flour
100g (4 oz) self-raising white flour
100g (4 oz) low-fat spread
50g (2 oz) granulated sugar
50g (2 oz) currants
1 × size 3 egg, beaten
75ml (⅛ pt) skimmed milk

Sieve the flours into a mixing bowl. Rub the low-fat spread into the flours until the mixture resembles fine breadcrumbs. Then stir in the sugar and currants. Make a well in the centre and pour the beaten egg and milk into it. Mix all the ingredients together well, stirring round in the well, gradually incorporating all the dry ingredients. Make 14 even-sized mounds of the mixture on a greased baking sheet and bake at 400°F/200°C (Gas Mark 6) for 10-15 minutes. Leave the Rock Cakes to cool on a wire rack before serving them.

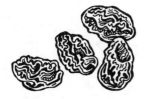
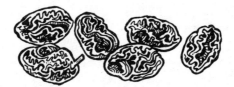

Maids of Honour

Makes 15-16

Pastry
100g (4 oz) wholemeal flour
50g (2 oz) white flour
pinch salt
50g (2 oz) low-fat spread
25g (1 oz) white polyunsaturated vegetable fat
a little cold water to mix

Filling
8 tsp pure fruit spread
50g (2 oz) low-fat spread
25g (1 oz) caster sugar
1×size 3 egg, beaten
50g (2 oz) self-raising wholemeal flour

Make the pastry by sieving the flours and salt into a bowl and rubbing the fats into the flour and stirring a little cold water into the mixture to bind it together. Refrigerate the pastry for 30 minutes, then roll it out and, using a 7-cm (3-in) round pastry cutter, cut out 15-16 shapes and put them in lightly greased patty tins. Put a half tea-spoonful of the pure fruit spread in the bottom of each. Cream the low-fat spread and sugar until the mixture is creamy, then fold in the beaten egg and flour. Put a small spoonful of the mixture in each case and bake them at 400°F/200°C (Gas Mark 6) for 15-20 minutes. Leave them to cool on a wire rack.

Madeleines

Makes 10

1×Victoria Sandwich recipe (see page 155)
75g (3 oz) reduced-sugar raspberry jam, warmed
100g (4 oz) desiccated coconut
5 glacé cherries, halved
angelica leaves to decorate

Make the Victoria Sandwich mixture as given on page 155. Spoon the mixture into 10 lightly greased dariole moulds so that they are ⅔ full and bake at 350°F/180°C (Gas Mark 4) for approximately 15 minutes or until the mixture has risen and turned golden brown.

Loosen the Madeleines round the edges with a knife and turn them out onto a cooling rack. When they are cool, thinly spread the jam over them and roll them in the coconut until they are coated in it. Put a glacé cherry on top of each cake and angelica leaves each side of it.

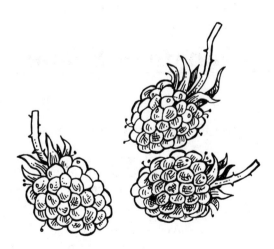

Jam Tarts

CHO 130g
Kcals 890

Makes 18-20

75g (3 oz) wholemeal flour
25g (1 oz) plain flour
25g (1 oz) low-fat spread
25g (1 oz) white polyunsaturated vegetable fat
2 tbs cold water
1 tsp polyunsaturated oil
6-6½ tbs reduced-sugar jam

Make the pastry by sieving the flours together into a bowl, rubbing the fats into the flours until the mixture resembles fine breadcrumbs, then adding the water and oil and working the mixture into a dough. Chill the pastry for 30 minutes before rolling it out on a lightly floured surface. Using a 5-cm (2-in) pastry cutter, cut out 18-20 rounds, gathering the scraps together and rolling it out again as necessary to use up as much of the pastry as possible. Put the pastry circles in lightly greased patty tins and put a teaspoonful of jam into each. Bake for 15-20 minutes at 400°F/200°C (Gas Mark 6). Cool them on a wire rack.

Cinnamon Scone

CHO 170g
Kcals 1100

Serves 8-10

225g (8 oz) self-raising wholemeal flour
pinch salt
2 tsp baking powder
3 tsp cinnamon
50g (2 oz) low-fat spread
1 tbs caster sugar
1×size 3 egg, lightly beaten
about 150ml (¼ pt) skimmed milk
1 tsp intense artificial sweetener

Sieve the flour, salt, baking powder and 2 tsp of the cinnamon into a bowl and rub in the low-fat spread until the mixture resembles fine breadcrumbs. Stir in the sugar then gradually pour in the egg and milk and stir the mixture until it forms a soft dough. Turn it onto a floured surface, knead it gently until it is smooth, then roll the dough out into a round approximately 18-cm (7-in) in diameter and 2.5-cm (1-in) thick.

Put the Scone on a lightly greased baking sheet and score it into 8 portions. Brush the surface with milk and sprinkle the remaining cinnamon over the top. Bake it at 425°F/220°C (Gas Mark 7) for 15-20 minutes until the scone has risen and is firm to the touch. Sprinkle the intense artificial sweetener over the scone once it comes out of the oven.

Rich Scones

CHO 210g
Kcals 1230

Makes 12-14

Same as in diabetic 'Home Baking'

225g (8 oz) self-raising wholemeal flour
½ tsp salt
50g (2 oz) low-fat spread
25g (1 oz) sugar
50g (2 oz) sultanas
1×size 3 egg, beaten with sufficient skimmed milk to make it up
to 150ml (¼ pt)

Sieve the flour and salt together into a bowl and rub the low-fat spread into them. Stir in the sugar and sultanas. Add the egg and milk, reserving enough to glaze the tops later. Knead the resulting dough lightly on a floured surface and roll it out to an even 2.5-cm (1-in) thickness. Using a 5-cm (2-in) pastry cutter, cut out as many rounds as you can, gathering together the scraps and rolling it out again to use as much of the dough as you can. Put them on a lightly greased baking sheet and brush the tops with the reserved liquid. Bake them in a hot oven at 425°F/220°C (Gas Mark 7) for approximately 10 minutes, then cool them on a wire rack.

Home baking

Curd Cheese Topping

Sufficient for a 18 cm (7 in) cake

75g (3 oz) curd cheese
liquid intense artificial sweetener to taste
flavouring and/or colouring (optional)

Beat the curd cheese until it is smooth and fairly soft. Add the sweetener to taste and colouring or flavouring if liked.

COOK'S TIP
Use the topping just to sandwich cakes together or to decorate the top as well.

Butter Icing

Sufficient for 6 small cakes

2 tbs powdered intense artificial sweetener
25g (1 oz) low-fat spread

Beat the ingredients together to form a smooth paste, shortly before you intend using it.

COOK'S TIP
This versatile icing can be flavoured in a variety of ways depending on what you like and the cake you are decorating. Try a few drops of vanilla essence or a tablespoon of cocoa powder or a teaspoon of coffee essence.

Festive occasions

Festive times need not be a time of denial. Try these tasty adaptations of traditional favourites and you'll be doing yourself good without you or your guests even noticing. You can feel confident that at Christmas, especially, a time when good food is at the centre of all the festivities, you, your family and friends can all enjoy a feast of *good* things — in all senses of the word.

Celery Boats

CHO 20g
Kcals 580

Makes about 24

1 head of celery, sticks separated, trimmed and washed
50g (2 oz) crunchy peanut butter
50g (2 oz) skimmed milk cheese
25g (1 oz) peeled prawns, chopped
50g (2 oz) reduced-fat cheddar cheese, finely grated
1 tbs mango chutney
twists of lemon, to garnish
paprika, to garnish

Cut the celery stalks into 4-cm (1½-in) lengths to make the 'boats'. Using a teaspoon, fill 8 of the celery boats with the peanut butter, 8 with the skimmed milk cheese, mixed with the prawns, and 8 with the grated cheese, which you have mixed with the chutney. Garnish each filled Celery Boat with either a twist of lemon or a sprinkle of paprika.

Note Because each boat is low in CHO they do not need to be counted.

Stuffed Iceberg Lettuce

CHO 20g
Kcals 370

Serves 4-6

1 Iceberg lettuce
175g (6 oz) skimmed milk soft cheese
1 tbs skimmed milk (if necessary)
1 red pepper, deseeded and finely diced
25g (1 oz) sultanas
25g (1 oz) walnuts, chopped
salt and freshly ground black pepper

Cut the top off the lettuce and reserve it. Using a sharp knife, scoop out the centre, leaving a 2.5cm (1-in) thick case. Chop the lettuce you scooped out and put it into a bowl. Then mix the soft cheese, milk, pepper, sultanas and walnuts together and season to taste with salt and freshly ground black pepper. Add half the chopped lettuce to this mixture and spoon it into the lettuce case and replace the lid. Put the Stuffed Iceberg Lettuce on a serving plate and garnish with the remaining chopped lettuce. Keep it chilled until you are ready to serve.

Broccoli and Mushroom Flan

CHO 110g
Kcals 1710

Serves 6-8

Pastry
100g (4 oz) wholemeal flour
50g (2 oz) plain flour
pinch salt
50g (2 oz) low-fat spread
25g (1 oz) white polyunsaturated vegetable fat
a little cold water to bind

Filling
225g (8 oz) broccoli cut into small florets
100g (4 oz) mushrooms, sliced
1 clove garlic, crushed
100g (4 oz) reduced-fat cheddar cheese, grated
2 × size 3 eggs, lightly beaten
1 × 150-g (5-fl oz) pot single cream
salt and freshly ground black pepper

Make the pastry first. Sieve the flours and salt into a bowl. Rub the fats into the flours until the mixture resembles fine breadcrumbs, then mix in a little cold water to work it into a dough. Chill the pastry for 30 minutes before rolling it out to line a 26-cm (10-in) flan tin or dish. Bake the pastry case blind for 10 minutes at 350°F/180°C (Gas Mark 4).

Meanwhile, steam or boil the broccoli florets until they have cooked through but are still a little crisp. Arrange them evenly over the bottom of the flan case, then sprinkle in the mushrooms and spread the garlic over the vegetables. Cover them with the cheese. Beat the eggs with the cream and season to taste with salt and freshly ground black pepper. Pour this mixture into the flan case and bake it at 325°F/170°C (Gas Mark 3) for approximately 45 minutes or until the egg and cream mixture has set.

Festive occasions

Prawn and Rice Ring

Serves 10

Ring
175g (6 oz) brown rice, cooked
275g (10 oz) frozen mixed vegetables, blanched

Dressing
4 tbs olive oil
2 tbs wine vinegar
pinch dry mustard
salt and freshly ground black pepper

Filling
2 tbs low-calorie mayonnaise
1 tbs tomato ketchup
few drops Worcestershire sauce
225g (8 oz) prawns
lemon twist, to garnish

Add the vegetables to the rice. Then combine all the dressing ingredients in a screw-top jar and shake it well. Stir just enough of the dressing into the rice mixture to make it glisten, then spoon it into a ring mould and press it down into it well. Chill it well.

Meanwhile, make the filling. Combine the mayonnaise, ketchup, Worcestershire sauce and prawns and stir them all together well. Carefully turn the rice ring out onto a serving dish and fill the centre with the prawn mixture. Garnish it with a twist of lemon and serve.

Salmon Quiche

Serves 6

Pastry
175g (6 oz) wholemeal flour
½ tsp baking powder
pinch salt
50g (2 oz) low-fat spread
25g (1 oz) white polyunsaturated fat
a little cold water to mix

Filling
1×200-g (7-oz) tin pink salmon, drained and flaked
100g (4 oz) cottage cheese, drained
2×size 3 eggs, lightly beaten
2 tbs skimmed milk
freshly ground black pepper
1 tomato, sliced

Make the pastry. Sieve the flour, baking powder and salt into a bowl, then rub in the fats until the mixture resembles fine breadcrumbs. Stir in enough water to bind the mixture into a soft dough. Roll the pastry out and line a 20-cm (8-in) flan tin or dish and bake it blind at 400°F/200°C (Gas Mark 6) for 10 minutes. When it has cooked, spoon the flaked salmon evenly over the bottom.

Now make the filling. Liquidize or blend the cottage cheese, eggs and milk until the mixture becomes smooth. Season it with freshly ground black pepper and pour it over the salmon. Arrange the tomato slices on top and bake at 400°F/200°C (Gas Mark 6) for 30-35 minutes or until the cheese, egg and milk mixture has set.

Mushroom and Onion Stuffing

CHO 40g
Kcals 490

25g (1 oz) low-fat spread
1 tbs corn or sunflower oil
100g (4 oz) mushrooms, sliced
1 onion, peeled and chopped
100g (4 oz) wholemeal breadcrumbs
1 tbs fresh parsley, chopped
salt and freshly ground black pepper
a little skimmed milk to bind, if necessary

Melt the low-fat spread and oil in a pan and lightly fry the mushrooms and onion until they have softened. Transfer the mixture to a mixing bowl and stir in the remaining ingredients, seasoning with salt and freshly ground black pepper to taste. Make sure the ingredients are well combined. Stir in a little milk to bind the mixture if necessary. Use to stuff a chicken or turkey.

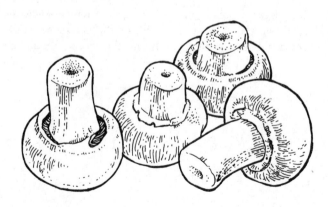

Bread Sauce

Makes approx 275ml/½ pt

1 onion, peeled and quartered
425ml (¾ pt) skimmed milk
6 black peppercorns
1 bay leaf
1 blade mace
3 cloves
100g (4 oz) fresh wholemeal breadcrumbs
pinch salt

Put the onion, milk, herbs and spices in a saucepan and bring to the boil. Remove the pan from the heat, cover it tightly and leave it to infuse for 15-20 minutes. Strain out the herbs and spices and return the milk to the pan once you have rinsed it out. Add the breadcrumbs and salt to taste. Simmer the sauce gently to reheat the milk, stirring occasionally. Adjust the seasoning to taste just before serving.

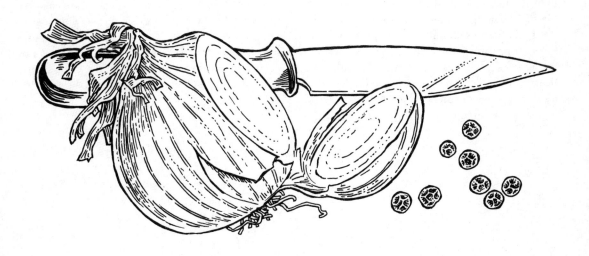

175

Christmas Cake

CHO 500g
Kcals 4360

Makes 36 portions

175g (6 oz) sultanas
175g (6 oz) raisins *-seedless*
100g (4 oz) currants
50g (2 oz) glacé cherries, chopped
275ml (½ pt) cold tea *(less if wholemeal flour not used ?)*
200g (7 oz) polyunsaturated margarine
50g (2 oz) ground almonds
275g (10 oz) wholemeal flour *(or ½ & ½)*
2 tsp baking powder
2 tsp mixed spice *or 1 spice mixed, 1 cinnamon*
3 × size 3 eggs, beaten
grated rind of 1 lemon *& zest.*
50g (2 oz) blanched almonds, chopped

use brandy/sherry as part of this!

add fruit

Put all the dried fruit into a bowl, cover it with the cold tea and leave the fruit to plump up overnight.

Cream the margarine and ground almonds until the mixture has lightened in colour. Sieve the flour, baking powder and mixed spice into a bowl and then gradually add the eggs and half the flour mixture to the creamed mixture. Fold in the lemon rind and chopped nuts. Carefully fold the remaining flour into the fruit mixture to make a soft dropping consistency. Pour the mixture into a greased and lined 20-cm (8-in) cake tin. Bake the cake at 325°F/170°C (Gas Mark 3) for 1 hour then reduce the heat to 275°F/140°C (Gas Mark 1) for a further 1-1¼ hours. Cover the top of the cake with greaseproof paper if it is browning too quickly. To test whether the cake is done, push a clean skewer into the centre, leave it there for 2 seconds and if it comes out clean, the cake is cooked. Leave the cake to cool in its tin before turning it out. To store the cake, wrap it in foil or leave it 1 day to mature and then freeze it.

Marzipan

This recipe makes enough marzipan to cover the top and sides of an 18-cm (7-in) cake.

100g (4 oz) ground almonds
50g (2 oz) caster sugar
25g (1 oz) white flour
1×size 3 egg

Beat all the ingredients together to form a smooth paste. You can do this by hand or use a food processor. Divide the mixture into two and wrap in cling film and store it in a cool place if you are not using it straight away.

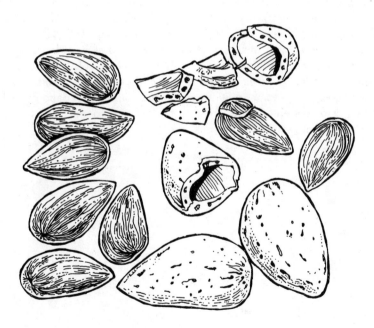

Festive occasions

Dundee Cake

CHO 340g
Kcals 2520

Makes 16 portions

175g (6 oz) low-fat spread
50g (2 oz) caster sugar
225g (8 oz) fine wholemeal self-raising flour
pinch salt
1 tsp mixed spice
3 × size 3 eggs, beaten
1 tbs skimmed milk — *omit if not using wholemeal flour?*
200g (7 oz) mixed fruit
25g (1 oz) split almonds for decoration

Cream the low-fat spread and sugar until the mixture is light and fluffy. Mix the flour together with the salt and mixed spice. Add the eggs to the creamed mixture, one at a time, with a little of the flour mixture, stirring and then beating the mixture thoroughly after each addition. Stir in the milk and beat again. Add the fruit and the rest of the flour mixture, folding them in lightly. Spoon the mixture into a greased and lined 18-cm (7-in) round cake tin. Arrange the split almonds on top in the traditional pattern of concentric circles and bake for 1 hour at 350°F/180°C (Gas Mark 4) and for a further 1-1¼ hours at 300°F/150°C (Gas Mark 2). To check whether it is done, poke a clean skewer into the centre of the cake, leave it there for 2 seconds and, if when you remove it the skewer is clean, your cake is done. Then leave it to cool in the tin on a cooling rack before turning it out.

Try cooking mid-oven on 3 (my oven) for ¾ hr. Then '1' for further 1¼ hrs. (Rec-rate oven. cooked cake in 1½ hrs.) See other recipes

Same as in Xmas cookery leaflet →

Mince Pies

CHO 170g 185
Kcals 1150 1260

Makes 12-16

Pastry
100g (4 oz) wholemeal flour
50g (2 oz) plain flour
50g (2 oz) low-fat spread
25g (1 oz) white polyunsaturated vegetable fat
a little cold water to bind

Filling
4-4½ tbs mincemeat
a little milk to glaze
a little powdered intense artificial sweetener *n granulated.*

Make the pastry by sieving the flours together, rubbing in the fats until the mixture resembles breadcrumbs, then stir in a little water to make a soft dough. Leave the pastry to chill in the refrigerator for 30 minutes, then roll it out on a lightly floured surface. Using a 5-cm (2-in) pastry cutter and a small star cutter, cut out an equal number of bases and stars. Gather the scraps together and roll it out again to use the maximum amount of pastry. Put the pastry circles in lightly greased patty tins and put a teaspoonful of the mincemeat into each. Place a star on top of the mincemeat. Bake the Mince Pies at 400°F/200°C (Gas Mark 6). When they are cooked, brush the stars with the milk and sprinkle a little of the sweetener over the top.

Festive occasions

Christmas Pudding

CHO 460g 465
Kcals 2920 3030

Makes 2×550ml/1 pt puddings; each pudding serves 12 each serving approx 20 CHO

200g (7 oz) wholemeal breadcrumbs
50g (2 oz) dark brown sugar
100g (4 oz) vegetable suet
pinch salt
1 tsp mixed spice
175g (6 oz) sultanas
175g (6 oz) raisins
100g (4 oz) currants
25g (1 oz) blanched almonds, chopped
1 medium cooking apple, peeled cored and grated
grated rind and juice of 1 lemon
1×size 3 egg, beaten
150ml (¼ pt) Guinness (stout) — Other recipes use brandy as alt.
about 5 tbs skimmed milk, if necessary

(Try halving ingredients - for just one pud.)

Mix the dry ingredients with the lemon juice, egg and Guinness, mixing them together well. Add a little milk if the mixture is too stiff. Pour the mixture into 2 550-ml (1 pt) pudding basins that have been lightly oiled. Cover them lightly with greaseproof paper and foil and steam for 2-3 [2½ - 3½] hours (or pressure cook at high pressure for 1-2 [1½ - 2] hours (consult the manufacturer's guide for your particular model). Cover the puddings with fresh greaseproof paper and foil to store them. When you want to reheat them steam for 2 hours.

Alternatives are from a similar recipe in "Balance".

Stuffed Dates

Makes 16

16 fresh dates
½ Marzipan recipe (see page 177)
16 petit four cases

Remove the stones from the dates, then fill each cavity with a little marzipan and put the date in a petit four case.

Easter Biscuits

Makes 28-30

100g (4 oz) low-fat spread
50g (2 oz) sugar
1×size 3 egg, separated and white beaten
100g (4 oz) wholemeal flour
50g (2 oz) rice flour
1 tsp mixed spice
50g (2 oz) currants
1 tbs skimmed milk, if necessary

Cream the low-fat spread and sugar together until the mixture is pale and creamy. Beat in the egg yolk then fold in the flours and mixed spice. Stir in the currants. If the dough is too stiff, mix in the milk to achieve a soft, pliable dough. Knead the dough until it is smooth, then roll it out on a lightly floured surface. Cut out 28-30 rounds using a 5-cm (2-in) pastry cutter. Gather the scraps together and roll it out again to waste as little dough as you can. Place the biscuits on a lightly greased baking sheet and bake them in the centre of the oven at 400°F/200°C (Gas Mark 6) for about 10 minutes. Brush the tops with the beaten egg white and return them to the oven to bake for about another 5 minutes. Cool them on a wire rack. When they have cooled, store them in an airtight container.

Hot Cross Buns

Makes 12 large or 24 mini

350g (12 oz) wholemeal flour
100g (4 oz) plain flour
pinch salt
1 tsp mixed spice
50g (2 oz) low-fat spread
15g (½ oz) sugar
1 sachet easy-blend dried yeast
75g (3 oz) currants
275ml (½ pt) hand-hot water
1×size 3 egg, beaten
1-2 tbs skimmed milk
scraps of pastry or flour paste, for the cross decoration
1 tsp sugar
1 tbs boiling water, to glaze

Sieve the flours, salt and mixed spice into a bowl. Rub in the low-fat spread until the mixture resembles fine breadcrumbs, then stir in the sugar, yeast and currants. Add the water and egg and mix to a soft dough. If the dough is too dry, add the milk. Knead the dough for 10 minutes so that it is well mixed and elastic, then put it in a lightly oiled plastic bag in a warm place and leave it to prove for about an hour. Knead the dough again and divide the mixture into 12 buns.

Put them on a lightly greased baking sheet and leave them to prove (covered) until they are light and fluffy. Make the traditional crosses either with thin strips of pastry or pipe them on with flour paste. Then bake them in a 425°F/220°C (Gas Mark 7) oven for 15-20 minutes, until they sound hollow when tapped on the bottom. Just before the end of their cooking time, dissolve the sugar in the boiling water and use it to glaze the buns while they are still hot.

Hot Fruity Punch

Serves 12

3 apples, cut into 8 pieces
3 oranges, cut into 8 pieces
12 whole cloves
2 cinnamon sticks
2 bottles red wine
550ml (1 pt) dry sherry
550ml (1 pt) unsweetened apple juice
1 orange, thinly sliced to decorate

Put the apple and orange pieces into a large pan with the cloves and cinnamon sticks and pour the red wine over them. Bring it to the boil and simmer, covered, for 10 minutes. Remove the pan from the heat and let it stand for 10 minutes for the flavours to infuse. Then, strain the wine and discard the spices, return the wine to the pan, pour in the apple juice and sherry and heat until the liquid starts to bubble at the edges of the pan. Pour the wine into a warm serving bowl and float the orange slices on top. Serve immediately.

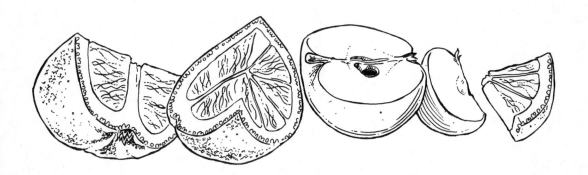

Festive occasions

Ideas for children

Children love to try different food, snacks, treats and drinks as much as adults do. As the majority of children are active and growing, it is even more important to provide them with healthy, nourishing meals. Quick food doesn't have to be junk food: why not try the American-style Hamburgers with the Bean Salad and home-made real Strawberry Milkshake?

You can make sure that there are plenty of protein foods in their diet by including meat, poultry, fish, dairy products, eggs and pulses. Vary what you give them and then you can be sure that they are eating a balanced diet and are less likely to become faddy eaters.

Sandwich Fillings

Makes 1 round

CHO 30g
Kcals 120

Skimmed Milk Cheese & Peanut Butter

1 tbs crunchy peanut butter
2 tbs skimmed milk cheese
salt and freshly ground black pepper
2 slices wholemeal bread

Combine the ingredients, mixing them together well. Spread the filling onto the bread.

CHO 30g
Kcals 130

Egg and Celery

1 egg, hard-boiled
1 stick celery, finely chopped
1 tbs reduced-calorie mayonnaise
2 slices wholemeal bread

Mix the ingredients together, combining them well. Spread the filling onto the bread.

CHO 30g
Kcals 200

Tuna and Mayonnaise

100g (4 oz) tinned tuna in brine, drained
2 tbs reduced-calorie mayonnaise
salt and freshly ground black pepper
a few slices cucumber and/or tomato
2 slices wholemeal bread

Combine the ingredients, mixing them well. Spread the filling onto the bread.

Welsh Rarebit

CHO 60g
Kcals 580

Serves 4

4 slices wholemeal bread
100g (4 oz) reduced-fat cheddar cheese, grated
pinch paprika
1 tsp mustard powder
1 tsp Worcestershire sauce

Toast the bread on one side under the grill.

Meanwhile, combine the remaining ingredients. Spread the cheese mixture on the untoasted side of the bread and grill gently for 3-4 minutes until the cheese is bubbling and golden brown. Serve immediately.

American-style Hamburgers

CHO 100g
Kcals 1270

Serves 4

450g (1 lb) extra lean mince beef
50g (2 oz) wholemeal breadcrumbs
1 tsp mixed herbs
salt and freshly ground black pepper
1 × size 3 egg, beaten
4 hamburger buns
4 lettuce leaves
2 tomatoes, sliced
1 onion, sliced

Put the minced beef, breadcrumbs and herbs into a bowl and mix them together well. Season to taste with salt and freshly ground black pepper, then bind the mixture together with the egg. Shape the mixture into 4 thick burgers and chill until needed.

Grill the burgers under medium heat for about 8 minutes on each side, or until they have cooked all the way through but aren't too dry. Then, split the buns and put a lettuce leaf and tomato and onion slices on the bottom half of each, put a burger on top then replace the other half of the bun.

Ideas for children

Stuffed Baked Potatoes

CHO 110g
Kcals 680

Serves 4

4 medium potatoes, cleaned
25g (1 oz) low-fat spread
1 onion, peeled and chopped
100g (4 oz) mushrooms, chopped
salt and freshly ground black pepper
1 tbs pickle
50g (2 oz) lean cooked ham, chopped

Bake the potatoes at 400°F/200°C (Gas Mark 6) for 45 minutes to 1 hour, or until the potatoes are soft all the way through.

Towards the end of the potatoes' cooking time, melt the low-fat spread in a pan and gently fry the onion and mushrooms. Season to taste with salt and freshly ground black pepper and stir in the pickle and ham. Cut the potatoes in half lengthways and scoop out the cooked flesh into a bowl, making sure that you do not pierce the skins. Mash it well, beat in the mushroom mixture, then spoon it back into the potato skins and return them to the oven, baking them for 10-15 more minutes.

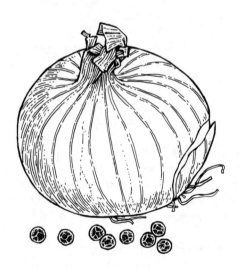

Pizza

Serves 4-6

Base
225g (8 oz) wholemeal self-raising flour
1 tsp baking powder
pinch salt
25g (1 oz) low-fat spread
25g (1 oz) reduced-fat cheddar, grated
150ml (¼ pt) skimmed milk

Topping
2tbs tomato purée
1 onion, peeled and finely chopped
pinch dried mixed herbs
50g (2 oz) button mushrooms, sliced
50g (2 oz) reduced-fat cheddar, grated

Sieve the flour and baking powder into a bowl. Add the pinch of salt and the low-fat spread and rub them in until the mixture resembles coarse breadcrumbs. Stir in the cheese, then add the milk and mix until you have a rough dough. Turn it out onto a floured surface and knead it until the dough is smooth. Roll it out on a lightly floured surface to form a 23-cm (9-in) round, then transfer it to a lightly greased baking sheet. Now add the topping. Spread the tomato purée over the surface, sprinkle the onion and herbs over the top, add the mushrooms, then sprinkle cheese over the top. Bake the pizza at 425°F/220°C (Gas Mark 7) for 20-25 minutes or until the cheese is bubbling and golden brown.

Bean Salad

Serves 4

1×439-g (15½ oz) tin red kidney beans, drained
1×200-g (7-oz) tin sweetcorn, drained
25g (1 oz) seedless raisins
1 small red pepper, deseeded and diced
1 tbs unsalted peanuts, chopped

Dressing
2 tbs olive oil
1 tbs wine vinegar
1 tbs tomato ketchup
1 tbs Worcestershire sauce
1 tsp intense artificial sweetener

Put the beans, sweetcorn, raisins and pepper in a bowl. Mix the dressing ingredients in a screw-top jar, shaking it well, then pour it over the Bean Salad and stir it until all the ingredients are coated in the dressing. Sprinkle with the peanuts over the salad just before serving.

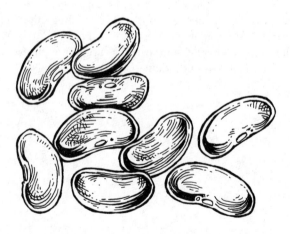

Ideas for children   190

Strawberry and Yogurt Jelly

CHO 10g
Kcals 90

Serves 4-6

1×packet strawberry-flavour sugar-free jelly crystals
1×150-g (5-fl oz) carton diet strawberry yogurt

Make up the jelly according to the directions on the packet and leave it to cool until it just starts to set, then fold in the yogurt. Pour the mixture into a wetted 550-ml (1-pt) mould or bowl, then chill in the refrigerator until it has set firm. You can turn the jelly out onto a serving dish if you want to — just dip the mould in very hot water for a couple of seconds, invert the serving dish and put it on top of the mould, then, holding the plate tightly over it, turn it quickly and then lift the mould off.

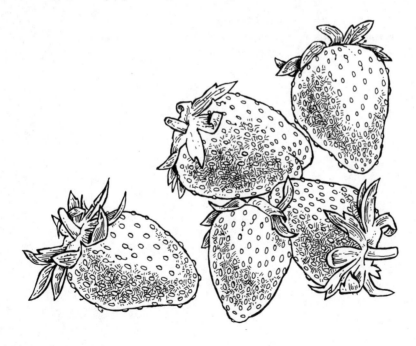

Ideas for children

Jelly Castles

Serves 4

1×packet orange-flavour sugar-free jelly crystals
4 tbs desiccated coconut
1×300-g (10½-oz) tin mandarin oranges in juice

Rinse out 4 150-ml (¼-pt) moulds or empty yogurt cartons with cold water. Make up the jelly according to the directions on the packet and pour equal amounts of the mixture into the wetted moulds. Cover them with clingfilm and chill until the jellies have set. Unmould the jellies into individual dishes, dipping them briefly into very hot water. Sprinkle the tops and sides of the jellies with the coconut and arrange all but 4 of the mandarin segments around the bottom edge of the jellies. Decorate the top of each jelly with a mandarin segment. Chill the Jelly Castles until you are ready to serve.

COOK'S TIP:
Use whichever flavour your child likes best and decorate with the appropriate fruit.

Pear Mice

Makes 6-7

1 × packet sugar-free jelly crystals
1 × 400-g (14-oz) tin pear halves in juice, drained and the juice reserved
18-21 currants
strip angelica

Make the jelly as per the instructions on the packet, using the pear juice made up to the amount given with water. Chill the jelly in the refrigerator until it has set.

Roughly chop the jelly and arrange it on a plate. Put the pear halves on the jelly, cut side down in a muddle — these are the mice! Press the currants into the fruit so that each 'mouse' has 2 'eyes' and a 'nose'. Cut the angelica into very fine strips and stick a few into each side of the nose to make whiskers.

COOK'S TIP:
This is ideal for children's parties and very easy to make.

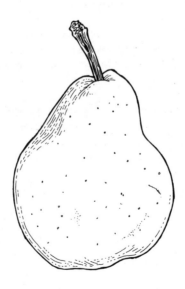

Ideas for children

Caribbean Drink

CHO 40g
Kcals 170

Serves 4

1 tinned pineapple ring, drained
2 small bananas, peeled
1 wineglass unsweetened orange juice
juice of 1 lime
½ tin (about 150ml/¼ pt) diet pineapple and grapefruit drink
about 6 ice cubes

Put all the ingredients into a blender or liquidizer and process until the mixture is smooth. Pour it into 4 glasses and serve immediately.

Peach and Ginger Fizz

CHO 30g
Kcals 130

Serves 4

2 medium peaches, peeled, stoned and chopped
1 wineglass unsweetened apple juice
1×500-ml (1-pt) bottle slimline ginger ale
crushed ice

Put the peaches and apple juice in a blender or liquidizer and process until the mixture is smooth. Add the ginger ale. Put the crushed ice into 4 glasses and pour out the drink. Serve immediately.

Strawberry Milkshake

CHO 10g
Kcals 120

Serves 2

275ml (½ pt) skimmed milk
100g (4 oz) strawberries, hulled if fresh, thawed if frozen
1 tsp intense artificial sweetener (optional)

Put the milk, strawberries and sweetener in a blender or liquidizer and process for 15-20 seconds. Strain the Milkshake into 2 glasses and serve immediately.

Useful addresses

United Kingdom
British Diabetic Association
10 Queen Anne Street
London W1M 0BD
United Kingdom
071 323 1531

USA
American Diabetes Association
1660 Duke Street
Alexandria, VA 22314
United States of America
1-703 549 1500
1-800 232 3472 (USA Only)

Australia
Diabetes Australia
QBE Building
33-35 Ainslie Avenue
Canberra ACT
PO Box 944
Civic Square ACT 2608
Australia
61 62 475655
61 62 475722

Austria
Österreichischer Diabetikervereinigung
(Austrian Diabetes Association)
Moosstrasse 18
5020 Salzburg
Austria
43 222 82 09 753

Belgium
Belgische Vereniging voor Suikerzieken
(Belgian Association for Diabetics)
BVS Secretariat
Charles de Kerchovelaan 369
B-9000 Ghent
Belgium
32 91 20 05 20

Canada
Canadian Diabetes Association
78 Bond Street
Toronto, Ontario M5B 2J8
Canada
1-416 362 4440

Czechoslovakia

Czechoslovak Diabetology Association
Internal Clinic ILF
National Diabetes Program
Coordinating Centre
762 75 Gottwaldov
Czechoslovakia

42 28235

Denmark

Diabetesforeningen
(Danish Diabetes Association)
Filosofgangen 24
5000 Odense C
Denmark

45 66 129006

Finland

Suomen Diabetesliitto r.y.
Diabetesförbundet i Finland r.f.
(Finnish Diabetes Association)
Diabeteskeskus
Kirjoniementie 15
SF-33680 Tampere
Finland

358 31 600 333

France

Association Française des Diabétiques
14 rue du Clos
75020 Paris
France

331-40 09 24 25

Germany

Deutscher Diabetiker-Bund e.V.
(German Diabetes Union)
Danzigerweg 1
D-5880 Lüdenscheid
Germany

49 2351 85053

Greece

Panhellenic Diabetic Association
Feidiou Street 18
Athens
Greece

30 1 362 9717

Hungary

Magyar Diabetes Társasgág
(Hungarian Diabetes Association)
Korányi S. utca 2a
Budapest 1083
Hungary

36 1 330 360

Ireland

Irish Diabetic Association
82/83 Lower Gardiner Street
Dublin 1
Ireland

363022

Italy

Associazione Italiana per la Difesa Degli
Interesi di Diabetici
Via del Scrofa 14
Roma
Italy

39 2 654 3784

Grand-Duché de Luxembourg

Association Luxembourgeoise du Diabète
PO Box 1316
Luxembourg
Grand-Duché de Luxembourg

352 474545
352 4411 1

Netherlands

Diabetes Vereniging Nederland
(Dutch Diabetes Association)
Puntenburgerlaan 91
3812 CC
Amersfoort
Netherlands

31 33 63 05 66

Norway

Norges Diabetesforbund
(Norwegian Diabetes Association)
Østensjøveien 29
0661 Oslo 6
Norway

47 2 65 45 50

Poland

Polskie Towarzystwo Diabetologiczne
(Polish Diabetological Association)
Kopernika 17
31-501 Kraków
Kraków
Poland

48 12 21 01 44
48 12 21 40 54

Portugal

Associaçao Protectora dos Diabéticos de
Portugal
(Portuguese Diabetic Association)
Rua do Salitre, 118
1200 Lisbon
Portugal

351 1 680041 (42)
351 2 682729

Spain

Sociedad Espanola de Diabetes
(Spanish Diabetes Society)
Colegio Official de Médicos
Santa Isabel, 51
28012 Madrid
Spain

341 2396519

Sweden

Svenska Endokrinolog föreningen
(Swedish Society of Endocrinology)
Department of Internal Medicine
University Hospital
S-75185 Uppsala
Sweden

46 18 663000

Switzerland

(Switzerische Diabetes) Gesellschaft
(Swiss Diabetes Association)
Hegarstrasse 18
CH-8032 Zurich
Switzerland

41 1 383 13 15

Yugoslavia

Savez Drustava za Zastitu od Secerne Bolesti
(The Association of Diabetic Societies of
Yugoslavia)
4a Dugi Dol
PO Box 958
41000 Zagreb
Yugoslavia

38 41 232 222
38 41 231 480

Further reading

Day, Dr John, *The Diabetes Handbook, Insulin dependent diabetes* (1st Edition), Thorsons, 1986

Day, Dr John, *The Diabetes Handbook, Non-insulin dependent diabetes* (2nd Edition), British Diabetic Association, 1992

Govindji, Azmina and Jill Myers, *Diabetic Entertaining*, Thorsons, 1990

North, Judith, *Teenage Diabetes*, Thorsons, 1990

Sönksen, Peter, Charles Fox and Sue Judd, *Diabetes at your fingertips* (2nd Edition), Class Publishing, 1991

British Diabetic Association

Diabetes affects just over two per cent of the UK population. Although it cannot be cured or prevented, it can be controlled by proper treatment. There may be times when you need advice or information and this is where the BDA can help.

The BDA is an independent registered charity with over 128,000 members and 400 local branches. It represents people with diabetes, liaising with Government Departments and professional bodies on matters concerning diabetes.

The Association provides information and practical advice for people with diabetes and their families. A wide range of literature, goods and videos are available on all aspects of diabetes including *Countdown*, a useful guide to the calorie and carbohydrate values of over 5,000 manufactured foods.

The BDA's magazine, *Balance*, is published every two months and is sent free to members or is available from newsagents. It keeps readers up to date with the latest medical news, local events and includes articles on living with diabetes. All diabetics have to follow a lifelong diet and *Balance* gives recipes and dietary information to help bring interest and variety to diabetic eating.

The Association also supports research to improve treatments and to find a prevention or cure for diabetes. Currently spending around £2 million each year, the BDA is the largest single contributor to diabetic research in the UK.

For over 50 years, the BDA has strived to achieve its aims, but it has only to be able to do so with the help of its members and supporters. Please join the BDA. For further details and an application form, contact:

British Diabetic Association
10 Queen Anne Street
London W1M 0BD
United Kingdom
Tel: 071-323 1531

Cakes – celebration 160
    cheesecake 148
    Christmas 176
    Dundee 178
    Fairy 156
    Rock 163
    Victoria sandwich 155

Breads: –
wholemeal p. 154
    158
tea
date & walnut 161

Index

Soups and starters

milk shake p. 195
mincemeat – see p. 179

Soups and starters